An Atlas of Investigation and Treatment
ISCHEMIC STROKE

For Laurie, Noah and Liora
        IES
For my husband, Rob, and the Stroke Team at Saint Luke's Hospital
        MMR

An Atlas of Investigation and Treatment

ISCHEMIC STROKE

Isaac E Silverman, MD
Vascular Neurology
Co-Medical Director
The Stroke Center at Hartford Hospital
Hartford, Connecticut
USA

Marilyn M Rymer, MD
Saint Luke's Brain and Stroke Institute
Saint Luke's Hospital
UMKC School of Medicine
Kansas City, Missouri
USA

Foreword by

Louis R Caplan, MD
Professor of Neurology
Department of Neurology
Beth Israel Deaconess Medical Center
Boston Massachusetts
USA

Special contributions by

Gary R Spiegel, MDCM (Neuroimaging)
Jefferson Radiology
Director of Neurointervention
Co-Medical Director
The Stroke Center at Hartford Hospital
Hartford, Connecticut
USA

Robert E Schmidt, MD, PhD (Neuropathology)
Professor, Pathology and Immunology
Washington University School of Medicine
St Louis, Missouri
USA

CLINICAL PUBLISHING

OXFORD

Clinical Publishing
an imprint of Atlas Medical Publishing Ltd
Oxford Centre for Innovation
Mill Street, Oxford OX2 0JX, UK

Tel: +44 1865 811116
Fax: +44 1865 251550
Email: info@clinicalpublishing.co.uk
Web: www.clinicalpublishing.co.uk

Distributed in USA and Canada by:
Clinical Publishing
30 Amberwood Parkway
Ashland OH 44805, USA

Tel: 800-247-6553 (toll free within US and Canada)
Fax: 419-281-6883
Email: order@bookmasters.com

Distributed in UK and Rest of World by:
Marston Book Services Ltd
PO Box 269
Abingdon
Oxon OX14 4YN, UK

Tel: +44 1235 465500
Fax: +44 1235 465555
Email: trade.orders@marston.co.uk

ISBN-13   978 1 84692 017 2
ISBN e-book 978 1 84692 595 5

Project manager: Gavin Smith, GPS Publishing Solutions, Herts, UK
Illustrations by Graeme Chambers, BA(Hons)
Typeset by Phoenix Photosetting, Chatham, Kent, UK
Printed and bound by Marston Book Services Ltd, Abingdon, Oxon, UK

Contents

Foreword

In neurology, *anatomy* is very important. Neurologists have a compulsive preoccupation with the anatomy of disease not shared by most non-neurologists, including general practitioners and internists. They are taught to ask not only *what* the disease process is but also *where* the abnormality is within the nervous system. The nervous system is made up of very different parts. Can one imagine body parts as different as the brain, spinal cord, peripheral nerves and muscles? Each component of the nervous system is very distinct and made of diverse subunits with different appearances, functions and susceptibilities to various diseases.

The brain is especially different from all other organs of the body. Most other internal organs are rather homogeneous. Parts of the lung, liver, pancreas, spleen and bone marrow all look alike and have identical functions. In these organs, disease is determined by the amount of the organ rendered dysfunctional, not by the location or 'anatomy' of the illness. A lesion in one part of the brain results in a loss of speech while a lesion very nearby could cause paralysis, loss of sensation, ataxia or many other functional abnormalities. The clinical symptoms and signs depend heavily on where the disease process occurs in the brain and on other aspects such as the size and extent of the abnormality and its nature (tumor, infection, vascular occlusion, hemorrhage, traumatic lesion etc.)

In patients with strokes and brain ischemia, anatomy is especially important. In order to effectively plan diagnosis and management, physicians will need to know not only where the lesion is in the brain, but *what*, *where*, and *how severe* the abnormality is in the blood vessels that supply the affected portion of the brain. They will also want to know if there are any additional abnormalities in other vascular structures. Heart and aortic lesions could be a source of embolism to intracranial blocked arteries. Vascular occlusions in other vessels could affect the body's ability to develop collateral blood flow to the affected region. Other arterial lesions could represent a threat for future strokes.

Stroke differs from many other neurological conditions in its timing. The term stroke indicates being suddenly 'stricken'. Doctors must act quickly to try to save brain tissue as brain ischemia is a medical emergency. "*Time is brain*" has become a familiar adage. In order to manage stroke patients, physicians must be very familiar with the anatomy of the blood vessels that supply the brain and know the types of vascular abnormalities and their predilection for different vascular locations. They must also be familiar with the various modalities that are able to provide images of the brain and the cervical and intracranial arteries and veins.

The good news is that advances in technology have now made it possible to image the brain and its vascular supply quickly and safely. Doctors can now rapidly determine the answers to the '*what*' and '*where*' questions if they are familiar with the anatomy, pathology and pathophysiology of brain ischemia and the technology available to show it.

Anatomy is visual: that is why the authors have chosen an atlas format to teach the fundamentals of ischemic stroke. This atlas is written by two very experienced active clinicians who are involved with the care of stroke patients every day. They succinctly and clearly review the basic aspects of anatomy, pathology and physiology, while illustrating the text with well chosen figures. The figures include anatomical drawings, pathology specimens and many images from modern CT, MRI, echocardiography and angiography. They emphasize the case method of teaching, since each stroke patient is different and their management depends heavily on the specific details of their condition.

I heartily recommend this atlas for anyone who cares for stroke patients. I suggest first reading the entire atlas thoroughly and then keeping it handy for review of and reference to aspects relating to individual patient scenarios. The writing is clear and easily grasped and the images are superb.

Louis R. Caplan, MD
December 2008

Preface

The paradigm for the diagnosis and treatment of stroke has undergone a revolution. It began in the mid-1970s when the first CT scans clearly differentiated acute hemorrhage from ischemia and proved clinicians right and wrong about the anatomical location and size of a stroke, and continued in the mid-1980s with the increased sensitivity of MRI. Then, in the mid-1990s, thrombolytic therapy for stroke was shown to be effective, and it became imperative that the diagnosis was correct and that patients were evaluated and treated urgently. The passive wait-and-see attitude toward acute stroke care was no longer acceptable. Stroke became a Level I medical emergency on a par with acute coronary syndromes and trauma. Interventional neuroradiology also evolved during that decade, providing catheter-based alternatives to vascular neurosurgery for the treatment of intracranial aneurysms and vascular malformations.

The modern era of stroke clinical trials was ushered in by studies comparing thrombolytic agents with placebo for acute ischemic stroke, carotid endarterectomy versus medical therapy, and antithrombotic agents for secondary stroke prevention. More recently, the treatment of aneurysms by neurosurgical clipping versus endovascular coiling, and neurosurgery for intracerebral hemorrhage and the malignant middle cerebral artery stroke syndrome have been studied. Now, catheter-delivered agents and devices, novel thrombolytic agents, and neuroprotective strategies, such as hypothermia, promise even longer therapeutic time windows and better outcomes. Advanced CT and MR neuroimaging are directing better patient selection for specific treatments and may also extend the window for revascularization.

These scientific advances have led to palpable changes in the way clinicians are trained and care is organized. Hundreds of hospitals in the USA are becoming certified as Primary Stroke Centers by the Joint Commission. Individual states in the USA are evaluating systems for organizing pre-hospital care. National organizations such as the American Stroke Association and the American Academy of Neurology are helping to promulgate quality measures and guidelines to improve and standardize the care of stroke patients. The US American Council on Graduate Medical Education has approved fellowship training in vascular neurology and interventional neurology, and the American Board of Psychiatry and Neurology offers vascular neurology subspecialty certification. There has never been a more exciting time to become an expert in stroke treatment and management. With aging populations and treatment options expanding, the need for stroke specialists is growing rapidly.

Our intent in this atlas is to introduce clinicians, residents in training, and medical and nursing students to the scope of neurovascular disorders. In this volume (Ischemic Stroke) and the companion volume (Hemorrhagic Stroke) we provide a practical visual guide to the emerging field of vascular neurology: neuroimaging and neuropathology organized around the major clinical diagnostic groups. This first volume addresses the evaluation of ischemic stroke, its diverse pathophysiology, and its emerging treatments. The companion volume introduces the causes of intracerebral hemorrhage, including intracranial aneurysms and the various forms of vascular malformations. We are unaware of any reference that offers this broad overview, and we hope that our atlas is an exciting stimulus for fellow clinicians and clinicians-in-training to consider joining our field.

Although the management of stroke and neurovascular care is increasingly driven by evidence-based medicine and formal guidelines, clinicians benefit greatly from the direct experiences of caring for individual patients so we have emphasized case studies.

Enjoy this atlas! The opportunity for effective treatment and improved outcomes for our patients has never been greater.

Marilyn M. Rymer, MD
Isaac E. Silverman, MD
December 2008

Acknowledgements

We are indebted to many physicians and other professional colleagues for their comments on the evolving manuscript as well as their contributions to the images included in the book. We would like to thank L. Christy Turtzo, MD, PhD, the first Vascular Neurology Fellow at the University of Connecticut and Gary R. Spiegel, MD, the lead Interventional Neuroradiologist at Hartford Hospital, for their critical review of certain individual chapters and Naveed Akhtar, MD, Interventional Neuroradiologist at Saint Luke's Stroke Center, for his review of selected chapters and images. Dr Spiegel contributed to the text, and assisted with the processing of innumerable angiographic studies.

Our sincere thanks to Robert Schmidt, MD, PhD, Professor of Pathology and Immunology at Washington University School of Medicine. Many of the beautiful pathology photos are his. We also had excellent assistance from Dean Uphoff, MD of the Pathology Department at Hartford Hospital and Louis R. Caplan, MD at the Beth Israel-Deaconess Medical Center in Boston. We are grateful to the following contributors from Hartford Hospital: Ethan Foxman, MD for neuroimaging, Inam U. Kureshi, MD, Vascular Neurosurgery, for intra-operative images of hemicraniectomy, and AVM and aneurysm surgeries, Paul Gaudio, MD of Ophthalmology, for retinal fundus photos and Cynthia Taub, MD of Cardiology, for echocardiography studies.

The strength of this project is based on the cases and neurovascular pathology that are evaluated on a weekly basis at the multidisciplinary Neurovascular Clinic of Hartford Hospital. Colleagues in this clinic are Donna Avanecean, Neurovascular APRN; Drs Kureshi and Spiegel; and in Vascular Neurology, Nora S. Lee, MD and Louise D. McCullough, MD, PhD.

The other chief source of case studies for this textbook comes from the inpatient service of the Stroke Center at Hartford Hospital. Core members not mentioned above from our stroke team are Dawn Beland, RN, Stroke Center Coordinator; Joao A. Gomes, MD, Neurocritical Care Medicine and Vascular Neurologist; Stephen K. Ohki, MD, Interventional Neuroradiology; Lincoln Abbott, MD, and A. Jon Smally, MD of Emergency Medicine; Michele Landes, RN, database manager; and our clinical trials coordinators, Martha Ahlquist, LPN, and Jennifer Blum.

The members of the stroke team at Saint Luke's Hospital were a great help in reviewing the work in progress. Irene Bettinger, MD, Charles Weinstein, MD, Steven Arkin, MD, Christine Boutwell, MD, Michael Schwartzman, DO, and Karin Olds, MD, are the neurologists, Naveed Akhtar, MD, is the neurointerventionalist and Debbie Summers, APN, is the coordinator of the stroke team.

A special thanks to Krzysztof Dzialo of the Radiology File Room, and Vladilen Bokotey, Radiology systems manager, both at Hartford Hospital. The input from these two individuals made feasible the digital manipulation of countless MRI, CT, and angiographic studies that ultimately form the heart of this textbook.

Finally, as a case-based, patient-centric endeavor, this atlas would not have been possible without the hundreds of stroke and neurovascular patients evaluated by our Stroke Center groups. Just as our experiences with the clinical presentation, morbidities and neurologic deficits, neuroimaging and neuropathology, and lives of these patients ultimately shape our growth as clinicians, we hope in turn to educate them about their disease and improve their quality of life. The rich breadth of this textbook is a tribute to these patients.

Abbreviations

ACA	anterior cerebral artery		INR	Interventional Neuroradiology/
AChA	anterior choroidal artery		IV	intravenous
ACoA	anterior communicating artery		MATCH	Management of Atherothrombosis with
AICA	anterior inferior cerebellar artery			Clopidogrel in High-Risk Patients with
AIS	acute ischemic stroke			Recent Transient Ischemic Attacks or
AMPA	a-amino-3-hydroxy-5-methyl-4-isoxazole			Ischemic Stroke (clinical trial)
	propionic acid		MCA	middle cerebral artery
AP	anteroposterior		MELAS	mitochondrial encephalopathy, lactic
BA	basilar artery			acidosis, and stroke-like episodes
BI	Barthel Index		MERCI	Mechanical Embolus Removal in Cerebral
CADASIL	cerebral autosomal dominant			Ischemia (endovascular device)
	arteriopathy with subcortical infarcts and		MRA	magnetic resonance angiography
	leukoencephalopathy		MRI	magnetic resonance imaging
CAPRIE	Clopidogrel vs Aspirin in Patients at Risk of		mRS	modified Rankin Scale
	Ischemic Events (clinical trial)		NIHSS	National Institutes of Health Stroke Scale
CHARISMA	Clopidogrel for High Atherothrombotic		NINDS	National Institutes of Neurologic Disease
	Risk and Ischemic Stabilization,			and Stroke
	Management, and Avoidance (clinical trial)		NINDS rt-PA	NINDS Recombinant Tissue Plasminogen
CNS	central nervous system			Activator (clinical trial)
CSF	cerebrospinal fluid		NMDA	N-methyl-D-aspartate
CT	computed tomography		OS	oculus sinister (left eye)
CTA	computed tomography angiography		PCA	posterior cerebral artery
DW-MRI	diffusion-weighted MRI sequence		PCoA	posterior communicating artery
ECA	external carotid artery		PFO	patent foramen ovale
EMS	Emergency Medical Services		PHQ-9	Patient Health Questionnaire (nine-item)
ESPRIT	European/Australasian Stroke Prevention in		PICA	posterior inferior cerebellar artery
	Reversible Ischaemia Trial (clinical trial)		PROACT-II	Prolyse in Acute Cerebral
ESPS-2	European Stroke Prevention Study 2			Thromboembolism II (clinical trial)
	(clinical trial)		PRoFESS	Prevention Regimen for Effectively
FDA	Food and Drug Administration			Avoiding Second Strokes (clinical trial)
FLAIR MRI	fluid-attenuated inversion recovery MRI		PT/INR	prothrombin time (international
	sequence			normalized ratio)
FMD	fibromuscular dysplasia		SAH	subarachnoid hemorrhage
GCA	giant cell arteritis		SCA	superior cerebellar artery
GE MRI	gradient echo MRI sequence		TEE	transesophageal echocardiogram
GOS	Glasgow Outcome Scale		TIA	transient ischemic attack
HD	hospital day		TOAST	Trial of ORG10172 in Acute Stroke
IA	intra-arterial			Treatment (clinical trial)
ICA	internal carotid artery		t-PA	tissue plasminogen activator
ICH	intracerebral hemorrhage		VA	vertebral artery
ICU	intensive care unit			

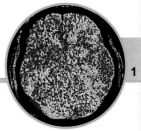

Chapter 1

Stroke Basics

Introduction

Stroke is the second leading cause of death worldwide and the leading cause of adult disability in many countries. It is imperative that all physicians understand the basics of stroke diagnosis and treatment for three reasons:

- Stroke occurs as an acute event, and people will access the closest medical facility or physician's office for help. Primary care and emergency medicine physicians need to be able to rapidly diagnose and treat patients with acute stroke symptoms.
- Emerging treatments for stroke are time-dependent. The earlier the initiation of treatment, the better the outcome.
- Once a stroke has occurred, the risk of a second stroke increases. It is essential that clinicians identify and treat the stroke mechanism and risk factors and institute medications (e.g., antithrombotic and blood pressure-lowering agents) when appropriate in order to prevent recurrence.

The goal of this atlas is to provide clinicians and students with a foundation in the clinical presentation, neuroimaging, pathology, pathophysiology, and treatment of stroke syndromes and neurovascular disorders so that they can make an accurate diagnosis and initiate treatment and/or seek vascular neurology consultation when appropriate.

What is a stroke?

A stroke is caused by a disruption in the flow of blood to part of the brain either because of occlusion of a blood vessel in the case of acute ischemic stroke (AIS) or the rupture of a blood vessel causing bleeding in or around the brain: intracerebral hemorrhage (ICH) or subarachnoid hemorrhage

(SAH), respectively (**1.1**). When stroke symptoms resolve and do not cause permanent brain damage, they are called a transient ischemic attack (TIA). Although the historical definition of a TIA is neurological symptoms lasting less than 24 hours, the duration of most TIAs is between 5 and 30 minutes, and can be considered a cerebral equivalent of cardiac angina.[1] Some healthcare professionals and patients refer to TIAs as 'mini-strokes,' but a TIA is actually a warning that a stroke may occur very soon.

Stroke epidemiology

Stroke incidence and mortality are increasing along with modernization and advancing longevity. Worldwide, 15 million people suffer a stroke each year. Five million of those die and 5 million are left permanently disabled.[2] It is estimated that by 2020, stroke mortality will have almost doubled as a result of an aging population and the future effects of current smoking patterns.[3]

Two-thirds of all stroke deaths and 60% of all strokes occur in low and middle income countries.[4] As infectious diseases and malnutrition decline in developing countries, stroke incidence rises due to decreased physical activity, increased tobacco use, and dietary changes. By 2040 there will be a billion adults aged 65 years or older at risk for stroke in low and middle income countries. In addition to the aging population, the major stroke risk factors worldwide are hypertension and tobacco use. In most countries, up to 30% of adults suffer from hypertension.[2] Men have a slightly higher incidence of stroke than women, but women have higher mortality rates. Black people have a higher stroke mortality rate than white people, and the mortality rate for Hispanic people falls between that of white and black people. There is a high incidence of hemorrhagic stroke in Asian people.[3]

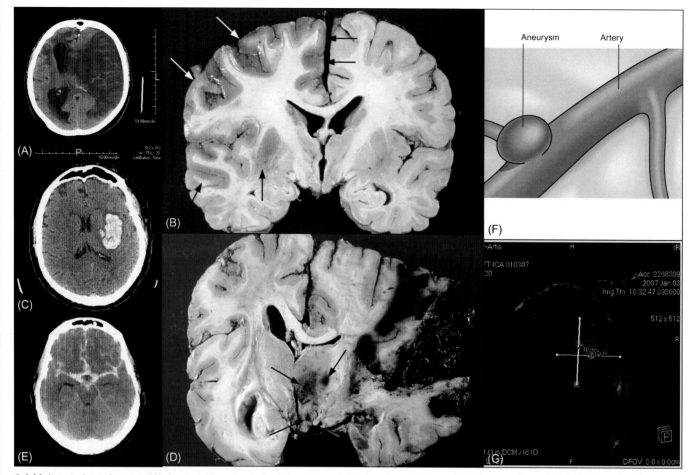

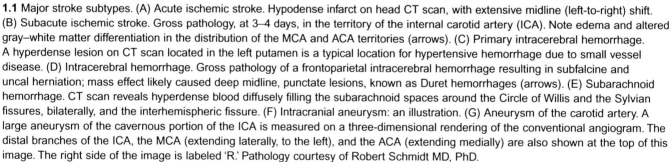

1.1 Major stroke subtypes. (A) Acute ischemic stroke. Hypodense infarct on head CT scan, with extensive midline (left-to-right) shift. (B) Subacute ischemic stroke. Gross pathology, at 3–4 days, in the territory of the internal carotid artery (ICA). Note edema and altered gray–white matter differentiation in the distribution of the MCA and ACA territories (arrows). (C) Primary intracerebral hemorrhage. A hyperdense lesion on CT scan located in the left putamen is a typical location for hypertensive hemorrhage due to small vessel disease. (D) Intracerebral hemorrhage. Gross pathology of a frontoparietal intracerebral hemorrhage resulting in subfalcine and uncal herniation; mass effect likely caused deep midline, punctate lesions, known as Duret hemorrhages (arrows). (E) Subarachnoid hemorrhage. CT scan reveals hyperdense blood diffusely filling the subarachnoid spaces around the Circle of Willis and the Sylvian fissures, bilaterally, and the interhemispheric fissure. (F) Intracranial aneurysm: an illustration. (G) Aneurysm of the carotid artery. A large aneurysm of the cavernous portion of the ICA is measured on a three-dimensional rendering of the conventional angiogram. The distal branches of the ICA, the MCA (extending laterally, to the left), and the ACA (extending medially) are also shown at the top of this image. The right side of the image is labeled 'R.' Pathology courtesy of Robert Schmidt MD, PhD.

Strokes occur at any age, but are more common in the elderly. Stroke risk doubles with every decade beyond 50 years of age, but 30% of strokes occur before the age of 65 in the USA.

Types of stroke

Ischemic stroke

Ischemic stroke, the most common type, is caused by an occlusion of an artery in the neck or in the brain, depriving a part of the brain of its nutrients, glucose and oxygen. The etiologies for AIS are diverse (**1.2**), and are reviewed in Chapter 2. The arterial occlusion is most often caused by a thrombus that has traveled to the brain (embolized) from a more proximal location in the body, such as the heart or from plaque in the wall of a proximal artery, such as the aorta or the internal carotid artery.[5] Less often, the etiology is a local thrombus developing immediately at the site of

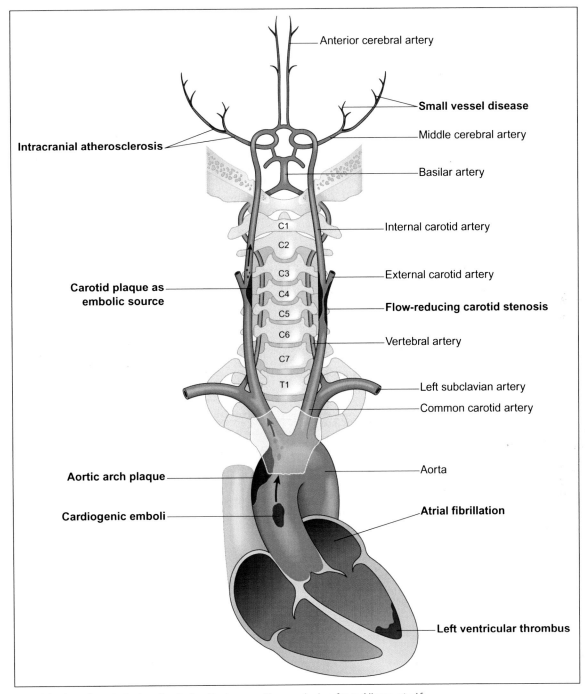

1.2 Common etiologies of acute ischemic stroke. Redrawn with permission from Albers *et al.*[5]

occlusion in large intracranial arteries (middle cerebral or basilar) or in small penetrating vessels, referred to as small vessel disease. Ischemic strokes account for 80–85% of strokes in most parts of the world, except for Asia, where ICH is more common.

Hemorrhagic stroke

ICH is caused by the rupture of a blood vessel, with bleeding directly into brain parenchyma, the ventricles, and/or spaces around the brain (**1.1C,D**). The rupture can occur because of acquired disease of the small penetrating arteries most commonly related to long-standing hypertension (small vessel disease), degenerative disease of superficial arteries (amyloid angiopathy), or from structural abnormalities of larger intracranial arteries, such as arteriovenous malformations. SAH occurs when an intracranial aneurysm ruptures and blood invades the spaces around the brain (**1.1E–G**). Aneurysms are balloon-shaped outpouchings of an artery where the vessel's wall has weakened.

Stroke symptoms

A general review of clinical symptoms is provided to help interpret information in the chapters that follow. (See the reference list at the end of this Chapter for textbooks that provide more detail on clinical stroke syndromes.[6–8]) The hallmark of stroke is *sudden onset of neurologic deficit*. Individual stroke symptoms depend entirely on what anatomical area of the central nervous system (brain, spinal cord, or eye) is damaged. Usually, stroke presents as a syndrome, a collection of symptoms that help the examiner localize the region of the central nervous system that is acutely injured.

1 *Headache.* Sudden severe headache is often associated with ICH and SAH, but is uncommon in ischemic stroke. An exception is ischemic stroke caused by carotid or vertebral artery dissection in which headache, facial, or neck pain are typical.[9,10]

2 *Weakness.* A sudden decrease in motor strength is the most common symptom of stroke.[11] The National Institutes of Health Stroke Scale (NIHSS) grading for motor strength (0–4) is a good way to reliably document the degree of limb weakness (*Table 1.1*).[12] Several terms are frequently used to describe stroke-related weakness (*Table 1.2*).

The degree of weakness usually depends on where in the motor system the lesion occurs. Peripheral cortical lesions may produce only focal weakness (paresis), most commonly involving the face and/or arm, or even the hand or individual fingers in isolation (**1.3A,B**). More proximal, subcortical or brainstem lesions usually cause a more uniform weakness of the face, arm, and leg on one side of the body (hemiparesis) due to the tight collection of motor tracts in those locations. Upper motor neuron lesions of the motor cortex may result in downstream atrophy of the motor pathways in the ipsilateral cerebral peduncle, called Wallerian degeneration (**1.3C**).

Table 1.1 NIH Stroke Scale (NIHSS) Score (www.ninds.nih.gov/doctors/NIH_stroke_scale)

1 Level of consciousness is tested by clinical observation, response to two questions and ability to follow two commands. 5 points
2 Best gaze assesses eye movements. 2 points
3 Visual fields. 3 points
4 Facial movements. 3 points
5 Hemiparesis and hemiplegia in upper and lower extremities
6 Each limb is graded individually (4 points for each limb)
• 0—patient can extend the arm (10 seconds) and leg (5 seconds) in the air without drifting downward. This indicates no weakness
• 1—patient can extend the extremity but there is downward drift; the limb does not fall to the table
• 2—patient can extend the extremity but the limb drops to the table
• 3—patient cannot extend the extremity against gravity, but there is volitional movement
• 4—patient cannot move the limb volitionally
The term paresis describes NIHSS grades 1, 2 and 3; and plegia describes NIHSS grade 4.
7 Ataxia is assessed in each limb (2 points)
8 Sensation is assessed on both sides of the body (2 points)
9 Language (presence of aphasia) is tested (3 points)
10 Dysarthria (2 points)
11 Extinction (formerly 'neglect') (2 points)

Table 1.2 Weakness associated with stroke

• Monoparesis: weakness of one limb
• Hemiparesis: weakness of both limbs on one side of the body
• Monoplegia: paralysis of one limb
• Hemiplegia: paralysis of both limbs on one side of the body
• Paraparesis: weakness of both legs
• Paraplegia: paralysis of both legs

Note: Paraparesis or paraplegia can result from ischemic or hemorrhagic stroke of the spinal cord, and rarely, bilateral anterior cerebral artery territory infarction.

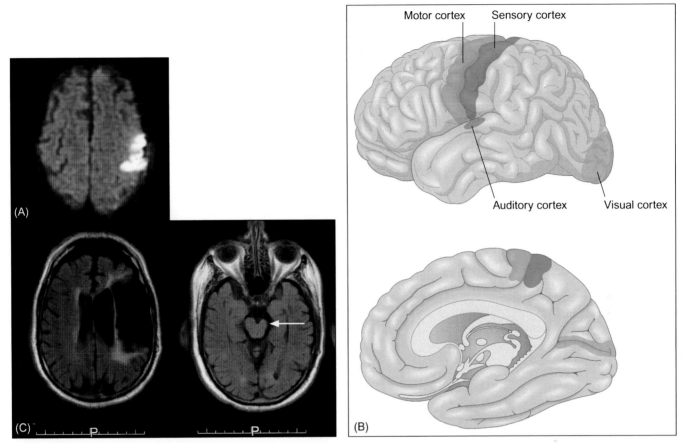

1.3 Hemiparesis. (A) Peripheral MCA infarction on diffusion-weighted MRI sequence, involving precentral gyrus (primary motor cortex). (B) Illustration of motor and sensory strips in the brain cortex. (C) Chronic left MCA-territory stroke, resulting in a wide region of encephalomalacia on the FLAIR MRI sequence (left). Atrophy of the ipsilateral cerebral peduncle (arrow), demonstrates associated Wallerian degeneration (right).

Most motor recovery from stroke occurs during the initial 1–3 months.[13] Incremental gains, however, can be made over the subsequent 9 months or beyond, and may depend on the availability of continuing rehabilitation treatment. Evolving concepts in neuroplasticity may offer hope for improved function years after the initial insult. Frequently, patients with mild residuae are left with minimal lower facial paresis, limited dexterity in the hand (e.g., diminished fine finger movements) and/or leg (e.g., diminished rate of toe tap), and/or foot drop.

3 *Ataxia.* Limb ataxia can occur with or without weakness and is a discoordination of movement usually related to infarction in the cerebellar hemisphere (**1.4**).[14] It is tested by evaluating rapid alternating movements and the finger-to-nose test in the upper extremities and the heel-to-shin test in the lower extremities. A midline cerebellar lesion may only cause mild vestibular symptoms and gait ataxia

without limb involvement. Long-term recovery from ataxia is usually excellent.

4 *Sensory loss.* Sudden loss of sensation usually occurs in association with weakness in the same distribution, but pure hemibody sensory strokes can occur, usually from occlusions of small vessels supplying the lateral thalamus, pons, or lenticulocapsular region deep in the brain.[15–17] The patient usually describes numbness and/or tingling paresthesias on one side of the face or the hemibody, a feeling often likened to 'novocaine in the dentist's office' or 'having a limb fall asleep.'

Cortical lesions causing sensory deficits are further dichotomized into those of the insular and opercular areas, affecting primary (primitive) sensation of pain or temperature with intact position sense, versus those involving the postcentral gyrus, resulting in cortical sensory loss affecting position sense, stereognosis, and graphesthesia (**1.3**B, **1.5**).[16]

Primary sensation is generally tested with a painful stimulus such as a pin-point or a stimulus of light touch, while cortical sensation may be assessed by testing position sense and by having a patient try to identify a number written upon the hand or an object placed into the hand. Inability to interpret the number written on the hand is **agraphesthesia** and an inability to identify an object such as a key in the hand is **astereognosis**.

Focal paresthesias, predominantly involving the perioral or finger areas (areas with strong representation within the homunculus), usually result from small distal emboli, to the postcentral gyrus (**1.5**).[16] Rarely, primitive sensory impairments evolve into dysesthesias, known as the **central post-stroke pain syndrome**.[16,18]

5 *Visual symptoms*:

• **Amaurosis fugax,** which is a term that describes transient blindness in one eye generally lasting 2–10 minutes, is a symptom of a retinal TIA often caused by an embolus from the ipsilateral carotid artery.[19,20] Permanent loss of vision in one eye frequently occurs when the central retinal artery is occluded, but this pattern of visual loss is generally not associated with other stroke symptoms (**1.6**).

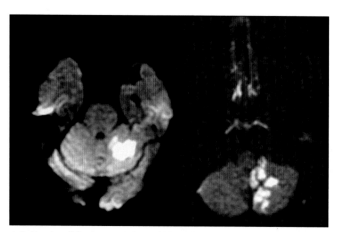

1.4 Ataxia. diffusion-weighted MRI sequences show (left) an acute infarct of the left cerebellar hemisphere, in the territory of the SCA, and (right) an infarct in the territory of the medial PICA.

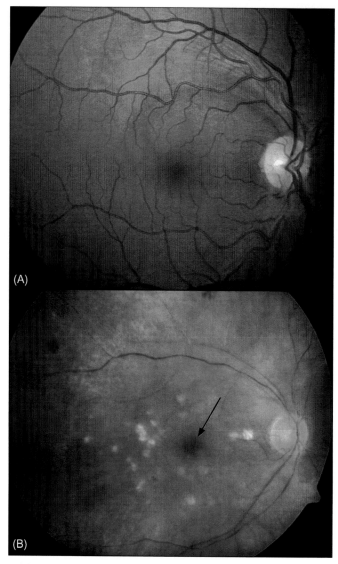

(A)

(B)

1.6 Monocular visual loss. A normal retina of the right eye is shown (A), contrasted with pallor and decreased vascularity due to acute central retinal artery occlusion (B). The diffuse whitening of the ischemic retina leaves only a 'cherry red spot' in the foveal center (arrow). (The small circular yellow spots are scars from past treatment of this retina with a laser.)

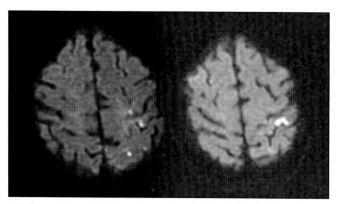

1.5 Cortical sensory loss. Cortical embolic stroke, involving the postcentral gyrus, caused a loss of cortical sensation. The emboli originated from atherosclerotic disease of the left ICA.

- **Hemifield visual loss** is loss of vision to one side involving both eyes.[21] It can be complete (hemianopia) or partial (quandrantanopia). It is detected by confrontational visual field testing in which the patient focuses on the examiner's nose and responds to stimuli in the fields of peripheral vision; it may be confirmed by computerized perimetry testing. Many patients with hemianopia are unaware of this symptom until demonstrated to them during their neurologic examination. Common presenting complaints are bumping into objects consistently on one side or, if driving, side-swiping a car present in the deficient visual hemifield. A stroke in the left hemisphere affecting the visual pathway will cause a right visual field defect, and vice versa. The further back the lesion is located in the visual pathway, the more homonymous (congruent) the defect in the two eyes (**1.7**). The chief practical results of a hemianopic visual field loss are that it usually precludes the ability to safely operate a motor vehicle and can make reading difficult. Spontaneous improvement of hemianopia typically occurs over the first 3 months post-stroke.[22]
- **Cortical blindness** is a rare clinical condition that results from infarction in both occipital lobes. The patient is blind but may describe visual phenomena. Anton's syndrome is the syndrome of cortical blindness in which patients deny their dense visual loss.[6]
- **Diplopia** (binocular double vision) may result from strokes in the posterior circulation because vertical and pontine gaze centers are located in the dorsal midbrain and pons, respectively (**1.8**).[6,23] The double images can

be horizontal, vertical, or oblique. Rarely, with brainstem stroke, the visual world may appear tilted.[6] When one eye is closed, there is no diplopia.

- **Forced gaze** to one side and gaze preference are important clinical findings in acute stroke.[6] Forced gaze means that both of the patient's eyes are deviated to one side and do not move from that position, a common early symptom in pontine strokes involving the horizontal gaze center. Gaze preference means that the patient's eyes are preferentially deviated in one direction but can be brought back to the midline or 'dolled' over to the contralateral side when the examiner moves the patient's head in the direction of the deviated eyes. These findings are consistent with a severe anterior circulation stroke involving the frontal eye fields on the same side as the gaze preference. For example, if the eyes are deviated to the right, one would expect a large stroke in the frontal region of the right hemisphere. The patient is said to be 'looking to the side of the stroke' (**1.9**).

6 *Visuospatial neglect.* Patients with infarction in the right (non-dominant) hemisphere are often unaware of the left side of the body or the left side of the space around them (**1.10**).[6,24] They do not recognize that the limbs on the left side are paralyzed or weak and are

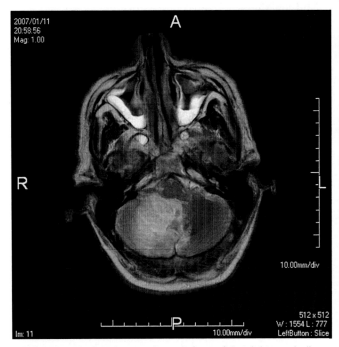

1.8 Oculomotor impairment. Acute infarct of the right cerebellar hemisphere, with mass effect on the brainstem resulting in diploplia (T2-weighted MRI sequence).

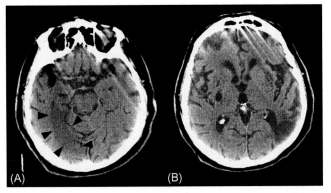

1.7 Hemifield visual loss. An acute infarct in the territory of the right PCA (arrowheads) on head CT scan (A) caused a left homonymous hemianopia. Other lesions, shown on a higher cut of this scan (B) in the right external capsule and the left posterior temporal lobe help explain this patient's vascular dementia.

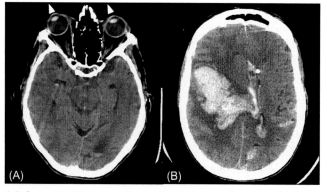

1.9 Gaze deviation. A patient with right gaze deviation (A). Note the far right position of the lenses of the eyes (arrowheads) on a lower cut of the CT scan. The responsible lesion, a large right frontoparietal intracerebral hemorrhage (B), impaired the patient's ability to drive the eyes to the left, a function of the right frontal eye fields.

often unable to identify their left body parts; the patient may deny ownership of a paretic limb. Most commonly due to right parietal infarction, this inability to recognize a deficit is called **anosagnosia**. In a milder form, when presented with visual or sensory stimuli to both sides of the body at the same time (bilateral simultaneous stimuli), patients may 'extinguish' (not perceive) the stimulus on the left. Hemineglect is a predictor for poor rehabilitation and functional outcomes post-stroke.[25,26]

7 *Language and speech production*:

- **Dysarthria** is slurring or mispronunciation of normal speech. The words and sentences are correct, but the patient may be difficult to understand. Dysarthria can be heard in patients with facial or tongue weakness and also occurs in strokes involving the cerebellum and brainstem. Patients often state that they are 'speaking like they were drunk.'

- **Aphasia** is difficulty with language processing: production and/or comprehension of speech. The stroke responsible occurs in the dominant (usually left) hemisphere.
  - *Broca's aphasia* (expressive and non-fluent) is a condition in which the patient has difficulty with naming and has very halted, frustrated, effortful speech. There is no difficulty understanding spoken language. The patient may state: 'I knew what I wanted to say, but just couldn't find the words.' Broca's area is an anatomical site at the base of the motor strip in the dominant hemisphere (**1.3B**, **1.11A,B**). This type of aphasia is often associated with contralateral limb (arm > leg) and facial weakness.

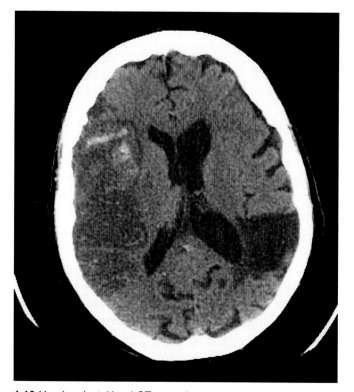

1.10 Hemineglect. Head CT scan demonstrates a subacute right hemispheric stroke that caused left body hemineglect. The evolving right hemispheric edema causes mass effect on the adjacent right lateral ventricle, while a chronic, left MCA infarct caused atrophy and associated *ex-vacuo* enlargement of the left lateral ventricle.

  - *Wernicke's aphasia* (receptive and fluent) is a condition in which the patient cannot understand spoken language, but talks 'fluently' in long sentences often devoid of nouns and most meaning. Wernicke's area is an anatomical site near the angular gyrus in the dominant hemisphere (**1.3B**, **1.11C**). Wernicke's aphasia may exist without motor impairment, and thus, the patient may be misdiagnosed as being simply 'confused,' or 'intoxicated.'
  - *Global aphasia* is the condition where the patient has both expressive and receptive deficits. Patients are frequently mute, and must rely upon visual mimicry to follow along with a neurologic exam.

Aphasia resulting from stroke will frequently evolve and usually improve, such that its basic characteristics fluctuate. Patients often will describe that their fluency will seem to break down when they are tired at the end of a long day. Subtle improvements in language-related deficits may occur even months to years following a stroke.

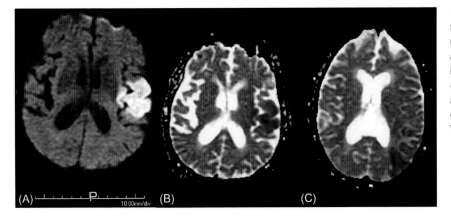

1.11 Aphasia. A diffusion-weighted MRI sequence (A) and apparent diffusion coefficient map (B) of a left MCA lesion, involving an anterior branch and affecting predominantly the insular cortex clinically expressed as Broca's (non-fluent, expressive) aphasia. A second acute left MCA infarct, apparent diffusion coefficient map (C) clinically associated with Wernicke's (fluent, receptive) aphasia.

8 ***Cognitive and behavioral deficits.*** Although aphasia and neglect are the most common higher cognitive deficits related to stroke, a wider range of neurobehavioral deficits include apraxia, memory loss and dementia, fatigue, depression, and other psychiatric disorders (e.g., emotional incontinence, anger, anxiety) can occur.[6,27] Given the advancing age of the general population, strong interest has arisen in the field of cognitive/neurobehavioral deficits associated with stroke. Large-scale clinical trials have begun to investigate vascular dementia resulting from multiple ischemic infarctions (e.g., **1.7**) and post-stroke depression.[28,29]

Stroke outcomes

An excellent predictor of stroke outcomes is stroke severity at presentation. A measure of stroke-related neurologic deficits, the National Institutes of Health Stroke Scale (NIHSS) score has been extensively studied in clinical trials and has been shown to be a very useful predictor of 3-month outcomes. NIHSS scores from 0 to 10 (mild deficits); 11 to 20 (moderate); and >20 (severe) have decreasing potential for good outcomes (*Table 1.3*).[30] The NIHSS is an excellent way for clinicians to communicate the severity of a stroke. Physicians and nurses caring for patients with strokes can be certified in the use of the NIHSS by the American Stroke Association or the National Stroke Association on their respective websites. Training materials can be obtained from the National Institutes of Neurologic Disease and Stroke (NINDS) website. The NIHSS score is heavily weighted toward anterior-circulation strokes, such that aphasia and hemiparesis often account for most of the points accumulated by any individual patient. Posterior circulation strokes frequently include neurologic

signs such as nystagmus, dysmetria, gait imbalance, or dysarthria, which do not contribute significantly to the NIHSS score, such that the score may underestimate the severity of a posterior circulation lesion.[31] In addition, a left middle cerebral artery stroke will have a higher NIHSS than an equally severe right middle cerebral artery stroke because of the scoring for language impairment. In practice, it is relatively simple to indicate to patients and their families how severe the deficit appears to be based solely upon the neurologic examination and NIHSS score. The potential for good outcomes is poor in moderate to severe strokes if left untreated.

Other common types of outcomes scales measure different dimensions of recovery and disability after acute stroke.[31] Some were developed specifically for stroke patients, while others look at disability and recovery following any type of acute brain injury:

Table 1.3 Admission NIHSS Score predicts short-term outcomes from acute ischemic stroke*

PROACT-II. Percentage of patients with minimal or no deficits (Modified Rankin Scale, 0–1), at 90 days post-stroke:

NIHSS 4–10: 63%

NIHSS 11–20: 24%

NIHSS 21–30: 7%

Adapted from Furlan *et al.*[37]

TOAST

NIHSS ≤6: 80% Excellent or good outcome

NIHSS ≥16: >85% Severe disability or death

Adapted from Adams *et al.*[30]

*Data derived from control groups' outcomes in two clinical trials, PROACT-II and TOAST.

- *Barthel Index (BI)* assesses activities of self-care and mobility.
- *Modified Rankin Scale (mRS)* assesses functional independence.
- *Glasgow Outcome Scale (GOS)* assesses general level of disability and recovery following acute brain injury.
- *PHQ-9*[32] assesses depression.
- *Stroke-specific Quality of Life scale*[33] assesses quality of life.

The National Institute of Neurological Disorders and Stroke Recombinant Tissue Plasminogen Activator (NINDS rt-PA) Stroke Trial combined the NIHSS, mRS, BI, and GOS into a single global outcomes measure.[34] Most acute stroke clinical trials use the mRS at 90 days as a primary outcome measure.

Diagnosis of stroke

The diagnosis of stroke is made by taking a careful history, performing a neurologic examination, and confirming the clinical diagnosis with an appropriate neuroimaging study. Seizures, hypoglycemia, trauma, and migraine are the most common mimics of the focal neurologic deficits in acute stroke. Brain tumors occasionally present with sudden onset of symptoms due to an associated hemorrhage into the tumor. Global symptoms of stroke such as altered level of conscious can be mimicked by metabolic encephalopathy. In most cases, the clinical diagnosis of stroke is not difficult. However, patients with global encephalopathy due to diagnoses such as venous sinus thrombosis, vasculitis, or multifocal emboli are more challenging; these cases are usually diagnosed by neuroimaging.

Neuroimaging

The evolution of modern neuroimaging has revolutionized the diagnosis and management of stroke. The modalities currently used are listed here and will be shown throughout the text.

- Non-enhanced head computed tomography (CT) scans are the most commonly available neuroimaging studies for acute stroke. This modality is excellent in detecting ICH and SAH (**1.1**C,E, **1.9**B), but is insensitive to small areas of infarction, especially in the posterior fossa (**1.12**). In most cases of early infarction (e.g., 1–4 hours after onset), the CT scan is normal. Subsequent scans over the next few hours begin to demonstrate an evolving infarct (**1.13**).
- Well-delineated hypodensity on CT indicates infarcted tissue (**1.13**C).

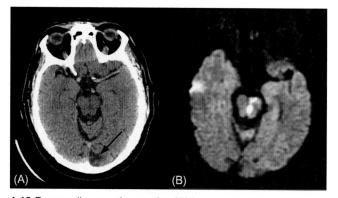

1.12 Paramedian pontine stroke. (A) Non-contrast head CT scan shows a faint hypodensity in mid-pons. The hypodense lesion in the left occipital pole (arrow) is likely a small, old PCA stroke. (B) The diffusion-weighted MRI study readily delineates the acute stroke as an area of restricted diffusion in the left medial pons.

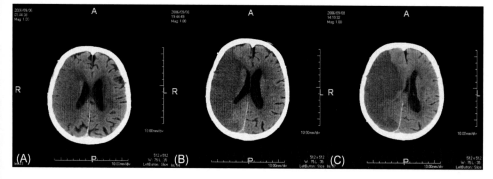

1.13 Serial neuroimaging, infarct in evolution. A right MCA-territory AIS on head CT scans. (A) Note blurring of sulcal spaces, and early hypodensity, at 6 hours. (B) The hypodense lesion becomes better delineated, at 24 hours. (C) The lesion demarcated as a wide hypodensity, with mass effect along the midline, at 40 hours.

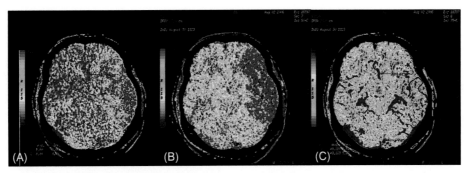

1.14 Perfusion CT imaging. (A) Cerebral blood flow map: hypoperfusion in a wide left-MCA distribution. (B) Mean transit time map: the region of slow mean transit time mirrors that of the cerebral blood flow map. (C) Cerebral blood volume map: no significant region of low volume is observed, suggesting that this ischemic tissue has not as yet infarcted. This cerebral blood flow/cerebral blood volume mismatch is consistent with an ischemic penumbra that might benefit from reperfusion therapy.[35]

- CT angiography using iodinated contrast dye can be used in the acute setting to diagnose large vessel extracranial and intracranial occlusions, and provides outstanding resolution for assessing the morphology of intracranial aneurysms and their position relative to the skull base.
- CT perfusion studies can delineate a region of decreased cerebral blood flow, and may be combined with other imaging modalities to identify hypoperfused 'tissue-at-risk' for infarction. If the area of decreased cerebral blood flow 'matches' the area of very low cerebral blood volume then that area will typically go on to infarct (**1.14**). If the area of decreased cerebral blood volume is quite small compared with the area of decreased cerebral blood flow (mismatch), reperfusion

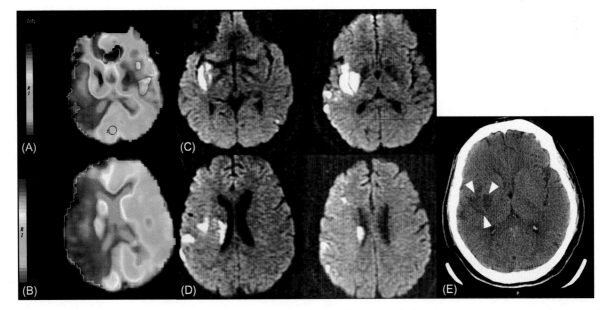

1.15 Perfusion–diffusion mismatch. This 52-year-old patient with a history of hypertension and tobacco use presented with acute-onset left hemiplegia, and a head CT scan (not shown) with a hyperdense middle cerebral artery sign, consistent with a proximal MCA occlusion. The perfusion-weighted MRI scan, here a map of mean transit time (A,B), shows deficient blood flow throughout the right MCA territory as a red region, but the diffusion-weighted MRI sequence (C,D) shows a smaller area of patchy infarction. This perfusion–diffusion mismatch directed reperfusion therapy, and the good outcome was confirmed with a follow-up CT scan 1 day later demonstrating only a small, predominantly subcortical infarct as a hypodense lesion (arrowheads) (E).

treatment may prevent infarction. The mean transit time also has predictive value.[35]

- Magnetic resonance imaging (MRI) is not as readily available for acute stroke diagnosis in many hospitals. The diffusion-weighted image sequence is sensitive to ischemia within minutes of the onset of symptoms (**1.4**, **1.15**). This technique is helpful when the diagnosis is in question and is excellent for identifying very small strokes causing minimal neurologic deficits. A 'dark' or hypointense lesion on the apparent diffusion coefficient map confirms that a diffusion-weighted magnetic resonance imaging lesion is due to infarction (**1.11**).

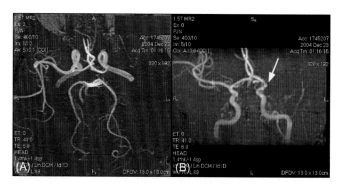

1.16 Magnetic resonance angiography, intracranial study. Proximal occlusion of the left middle cerebral artery, the M1 segment, on coronal (A) and transaxial (B) views (arrow). No distal, left hemispheric blood flow is observed.

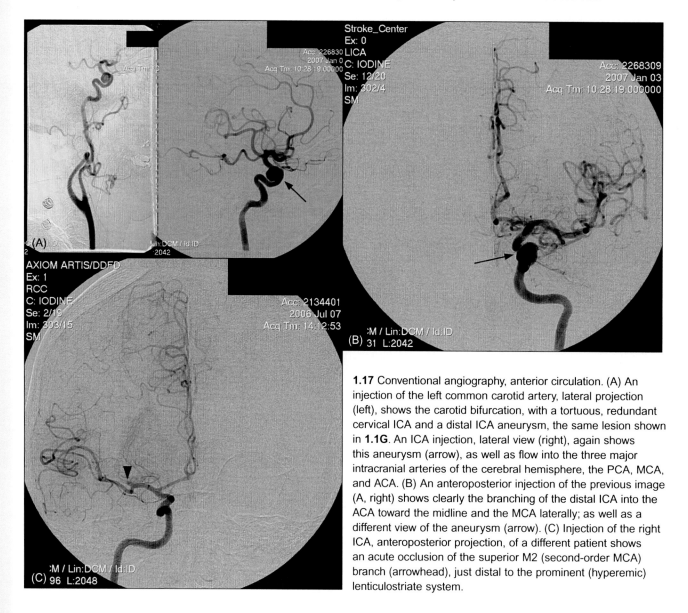

1.17 Conventional angiography, anterior circulation. (A) An injection of the left common carotid artery, lateral projection (left), shows the carotid bifurcation, with a tortuous, redundant cervical ICA and a distal ICA aneurysm, the same lesion shown in **1.1G**. An ICA injection, lateral view (right), again shows this aneurysm (arrow), as well as flow into the three major intracranial arteries of the cerebral hemisphere, the PCA, MCA, and ACA. (B) An anteroposterior injection of the previous image (A, right) shows clearly the branching of the distal ICA into the ACA toward the midline and the MCA laterally; as well as a different view of the aneurysm (arrow). (C) Injection of the right ICA, anteroposterior projection, of a different patient shows an acute occlusion of the superior M2 (second-order MCA) branch (arrowhead), just distal to the prominent (hyperemic) lenticulostriate system.

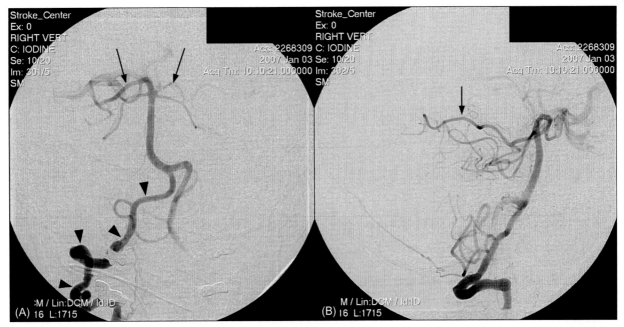

1.18 Conventional angiography, posterior circulation. (A) A right vertebral artery (arrowheads) injection, anteroposterior view, shows the major intracranial arteries of the posterior circulation. The SCAs course immediately below and almost parallel to the PCAs (arrows). (B) A lateral view of the image in (A) shows a slightly later time-frame of this injection, with the PCA (arrow) at the top of the BA extending posteriorly toward the occipital lobe.

- When there is a small area of abnormality in the diffusion-weighted image sequence and a large area of abnormality in the perfusion-weighted sequence, there is a so-called 'perfusion/diffusion mismatch' (**1.15**),[36] which is akin to the cerebral blood flow/cerebral blood volume findings of perfusion CT imaging. A mismatch indicates an opportunity to salvage tissue that is underperfused but not yet showing a diffusion deficit indicating cellular injury. This kind of physiologic analysis may be the best way to predict which cases could tolerate a longer time window for intravenous reperfusion therapy and/or those who should go on to neurointervention.

- Magnetic resonance angiography is useful in screening for extracranial and intracranial large vessel occlusions or stenoses (**1.16**). In general, magnetic resonance angiography tends to overestimate the degree of stenosis, but gadolinium, a contrast agent, improves the quality of this technique.

- Digital subtraction angiography, also called conventional cerebral angiography (**1.17, 1.18**), is the gold standard for visualization of extracranial and intracranial vessels, but has the disadvantage of being invasive and requiring specialized equipment, technicians, and interventional neuroradiologists.

References

1. Johnston S. Transient ischemic attack. *N Engl J Med* 2002; **347**: 1687–92.

2. UN Chronicle Health Watch. *Atlas of Heart Disease and Stroke*. 2005; **0105**: 46.

3. Warlow C, Sudlow C, Dennis M, Wardlaw J, Sandercock P. Stroke. *Lancet* 2003; **362**: 1211–24.

4. Reddy K, Yusuf S. Emerging epidemic of cardiovascular disease in developing countries. *Circulation* 1998; **97**: 596–601.

5. Albers G, Amarenco P, Easton J, Sacco R, Teal P. Antithrombotic and thrombolytic therapy for ischemic stroke: The Seventh ACCP Conference on Antithrombotic and Thrombolytic Therapy. *Chest* 2004; **3**: S483–512.

6. Brazis P, Masdeu J, Biller J. *Localization in Clinical Neurology*, 4th edn. Philadelphia: Lippincott Williams & Wilkins; 2001.

7. Bogousslavsky J, Hommel M. Ischemic stroke syndromes: clinical features, anatomy, vascular territories. In: Adams H, Jr, ed. *Handbook of Cerebrovascular Diseases*. New York: Marcel Dekker; 1993: 51–94.

8. Bogousslavsky J, Caplan L. *Stroke Syndromes*, 2nd edn. New York: Cambridge University Press; 2001.

9. Estol C. Headache: stroke symptoms and signs. In: Bogousslavsky J, Caplan L, eds. *Stroke Syndromes*, 2nd edn. New York: Cambridge University Press; 2001: 60–75.

10. Schievink W. Spontaneous dissection of the carotid and vertebral arteries. *N Engl J Med* 2001; **344**: 898–906.

11. Pinho e Melo T, Bogousslavsky J. Hemiparesis and other types of motor weakness. In: Bogousslavsky J, Caplan L, eds. *Stroke Syndromes*, 2nd edn. New York: Cambridge University Press; 2001: 22–33.

12. Goldstein L, Bertels C, Davis J. Interrater reliability of the NIH stroke scale. *Arch Neurol* 1989; **46**: 660–2.

13. Dobkin B. Rehabilitation after stroke. *N Engl J Med* 2005; **352**: 1677–84.

14. Timmann D, Diener H. Cerebellar ataxia. In: Bogousslavsky J, Caplan L, eds. *Stroke Syndromes*, 2nd edn. New York: Cambridge University Press; 2001: 48–59.

15. Kim J. Sensory abnormality. In: Bogousslavsky J, Caplan L, eds. *Stroke Syndromes*, 2nd edn. New York: Cambridge University Press; 2001.

16. Kim J. Patterns of sensory abnormality in cortical stroke: evidence for a dichotomized sensory system. *Neurology* 2007; **68**: 174–80.

17. Schmahmann J. Vascular syndromes of the thalamus. *Stroke* 2003; **34**: 2264–78.

18. Bowsher D, Leijon G, Thuomas K-A. Central poststroke pain: correlation of MRI with clinical pain characteristics and sensory abnormalities. *Neurology* 1998; **51**: 1352–8.

19. Benavente O, Eliasziw M, Streifler J, *et al.* Prognosis after transient monocular blindness associated with carotid-artery stenosis. *N Engl J Med* 2001; **345**: 1084–90.

20. Wray S. Visual symptoms (eye). In: Bogousslavsky J, Caplan L, eds. *Stroke Syndromes*, 2nd edn. New York: Cambridge University Press; 2001: 111–28.

21. Barton J, Caplan L. Cerebral visual dysfunction. In: Bogousslavsky J, Caplan L, eds. *Stroke Syndromes*, 2nd edn. New York: Cambridge University Press; 2001: 87–110.

22. Zhang X, Kedar S, Lynn M, Newman N, Biousse V. Natural history of homonymous hemianopia. *Neurology* 2006; **66**: 901–5.

23. Pierrot-Deseilligny C. Eye movement abnormalities. In: Bogousslavsky J, Caplan L, eds. *Stroke Syndromes*, 2nd edn. New York: Cambridge University Press; 2001: 76–86.

24. Clarke S. Right hemisphere syndromes. In: Bogousslavsky J, Caplan L, eds. *Stroke Syndromes*, 2nd edn. New York: Cambridge University Press; 2001: 264–72.

25. Beis J-M, Keller C, Morin N, *et al.* Right spatial neglect after left hemisphere stroke: a qualitative and quantitative study. *Neurology* 2004; **63**: 1600–5.

26. Buxbaum L, Ferraro M, Veramonti T, *et al.* Hemispatial neglect: subtypes, neuroanatomy, and disability. *Neurology* 2004; **62**: 749–56.

27. Bogousslavsky J. William Feinberg Lecture 2002: emotions, mood, and behavior after stroke. *Stroke* 2003; **34**: 1046–50.

28. Hackett M, Anderson C, House A. Management of depression after stroke: a systematic review of pharmacological therapies. *Stroke* 2005; **36**: 1092–7.

29. Erkinjuntti T, Roman G, Gauthier S, Feldman H, Rockwood K. Emerging therapies for vascular dementia and vascular cognitive impairment. *Stroke* 2004; **35**: 1010–17.

30. Adams HP Jr, Davis P, Leira E, *et al.* Baseline NIH Stroke Scale score strongly predicts outcome after stroke: a report of the Trial of Org 10172 in Acute Stroke Treatment (TOAST). *Neurology* 1999; **53**: 126–31.

31. Kasner S. Clinical interpretation and use of stroke scales. *Lancet Neurol* 2006; **5**: 603–12.

32. Williams L, Brizendine E, Plue L, *et al.* Performance of the PHQ-9 as a screening tool for depression after stroke. *Stroke* 2005; **36**: 635–8.

33. Williams L, Weinberger M, Harris L, Clark D, Biller J. Development of a stroke-specific quality of life scale. *Stroke* 1999; **30**: 1362–9.

34. National Institute of Neurological Disorders and Stroke rt-PA Stroke Study Group. Tissue plasminogen activator for acute ischemic stroke. *N Engl J Med* 1995; **333**: 1581–7.

35. Wintermark M, Reichart M, Thiran J-P, *et al.* Prognostic accuracy of cerebral blood flow measurement by perfusion computed tomography, at the time of emergency room admission in acute stroke patients. *Ann Neurol* 2002; 51: 417–32.

36. Davalos A, Blanco M, Pedraza S, *et al.* The clinical–DWI mismatch: A new diagnostic approach to the brain tissue at risk of infarction. *Neurology* 2004; **62**: 2187–92.

37. Furlan A, Higashida R, Katzan I, Abou–Chebl A. Intra-arterial thrombolysis in acute ischemic stroke. In: Lyden P, ed. *Thrombolytic Therapy for Stroke*. Totowa, NJ: Humana Press; 2001: 175–95.

Further reading

Bogousslavsky J, Caplan LR. *Stroke Syndromes*, 2nd edn. New York: Cambridge University Press; 2001.

Brazis PW, Masdeu JC, Biller J. *Localization in Clinical Neurology*, 4th edn. New York: Little, Brown and Company; 2001.

Kasner S. Clinical interpretation and use of stroke scales. *Lancet Neurol* 2006; **5**: 603–12.

Resources for patients

American Stroke Association: http://www.strokeassociation.org

National Stroke Association: http://www.stroke.org

Chapter 2

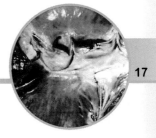

Pathophysiology

Introduction

Ischemic strokes can be classified by anatomic location and by pathophysiologic mechanism. A stroke in the distribution of the middle cerebral artery (MCA; arterial territory: *anatomic location*) could be caused by an embolus originating from the heart (cardioembolic source: *pathophysiologic mechanism*). Both types of stroke classifications are important to understand. The symptoms of ischemic stroke (Chapter 1) are entirely dependent upon the arterial territory involved (Chapters 3 and 4). The current chapter addresses the diverse pathophysiology of ischemic stroke.

Stroke pathophysiology is inferred from the patient's medical history, diagnostic work-up, and the pattern and location of the stroke on neuroimaging. It is critical for the clinician to identify the pathophysiologic mechanism, because the probable cause of the stroke informs the medications and procedures employed for secondary stroke prevention. For example, a patient with an ischemic stroke in the MCA territory presenting with new-onset atrial fibrillation and no other apparent source of thromboembolism likely has a cardiogenic source, and should be started on an anticoagulant such as warfarin.

The pathophysiologic classification system described originally in the TOAST (Trial of ORG 10172 in Acute Stroke Treatment) clinical trial has become the standard for vascular neurology (*Table 2.1*).[1,2] The percentages noted for each classification discussed below are approximate and vary by the population and registry data studied.

Large vessel disease (atherosclerosis)

Large vessel atherosclerotic disease accounts for 30–40% of ischemic strokes. This category includes atherosclerotic disease in the aorta, and major extracranial and intracranial

Table 2.1 TOAST criteria[1]

1. Large vessel disease (atherosclerosis)
2. Cardiac source (cardioembolic)
3. Small vessel disease (arteriolosclerosis; 'lacunar syndromes')
4. Other determined etiology
5. Undetermined etiology

arteries (**2.1**). Thrombosis can develop locally at the site of arterial disease, or the diseased arterial segment can be a source of embolism to a more distal segment or branch of the artery. The latter circumstance, artery-to-artery embolism, is most commonly observed when atherosclerotic plaque located at the proximal internal carotid artery (ICA) embolizes to the MCA.

The most common sites of atherosclerotic disease are the aortic arch, carotid artery bifurcation, origins of the vertebral and common carotid arteries , the proximal (M1) segment of the MCA (case study 1), the distal vertebral arteries, and the middle and distal sections of the basilar artery. Intracranial stenosis occurs more frequently in Asian and black populations.[3] Intracranial MCA disease may cause stroke by several mechanisms: distal atheroemboli, borderzone lesions, and lenticulostriate perforator infarcts (i.e., branch artery occlusion) (**case study 1**).

The diagnosis of large vessel disease is made by imaging the blood vessels with CT angiography, MRA, ultrasound, conventional angiography, and transesophageal echocardiography. This last modality enables visualization of atherosclerotic plaque within the aorta (**2.1C,D**).[4] Plaque thickness >4 mm has been associated with a heightened risk for aortoembolic ischemic stroke.[5]

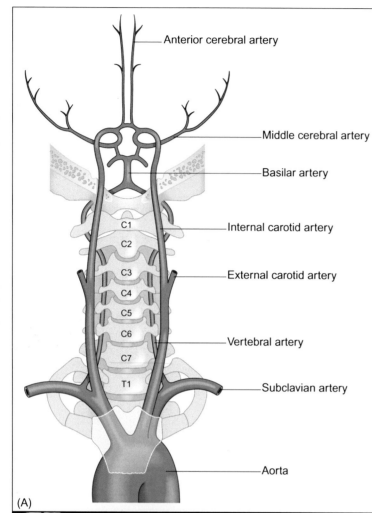

Anterior cerebral artery

Middle cerebral artery

Basilar artery

C1

Internal carotid artery

C2

C3

External carotid artery

C4

C5

C6

Vertebral artery

C7

T1

Subclavian artery

Aorta

(A)

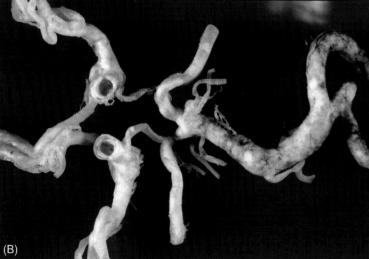

(B)

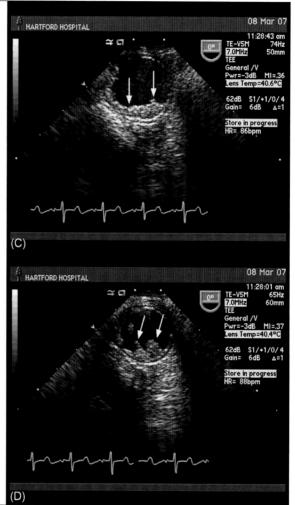

(C)

(D)

2.1 Large vessel disease. Illustration of the major cervical arteries supplying the brain (A). The common carotid arteries branch into the external and internal carotid arteries. The vertebral arteries course through the transverse foramina of the C6 through C1 vertebral bodies. Adapted with permission from Osborn.[20] The circle of Willis (B): Gross pathology demonstrates widespread large vessel atherosclerosis, recognized by heterogeneous plaque in the arterial walls. Transesophageal echocardiography: non-mobile (C) and mobile (D) components of atherosclerotic plaque (arrows) shown as a thickness in the wall of the aorta, on transverse images. The mobile plaque is heterogeneous and irregular, protruding into the lumen (arrows). Echocardiography courtesy of Cynthia Taub, MD.

Cardioembolic disease (cardiac source of emboli)

Cardioembolic disease accounts for about 25% of ischemic strokes (**case study 2**). Atrial fibrillation is, by far, the most common cause of cardioembolic stroke.[6] Cardiac sources of emboli causing stroke are stratified by major and minor risk (**2.2**; *Table 2.2*).[7] Congenital heart conditions with right-to-left shunt, such as patent foramen ovale (**2.3**) or atrial septal aneurysms, are less frequent causes of cardiogenic emboli.[8]

The diagnosis of these conditions is made through standard electrocardiography, cardiac monitoring, and echocardiography. Transesophageal echocardiography (TEE) is more sensitive than is transthoracic echocardiography for identifying atrial septal aneurysm and defect, patent foramen ovale,

atrial myxoma, atrial thrombus, atrial appendage thrombus, aortic arch atheromas, and mitral valve vegetations (**2.2**).[7,9]

Small vessel disease (arteriolosclerosis)

Arteriolosclerosis accounts for 20% of ischemic strokes. The lesions are small 'lacunes' deep in the brain referred to as 'lacunar infarcts.'[10] Local occlusions of small penetrating end-arteries, such as the lenticulostriate branches of the MCA, the thalamostriate branches of the posterior cerebral artery, and the pontine perforators from the basilar artery, are the cause (**2.4A**). Typically, patients with small vessel disease have one or more of the classic cardiovascular risk factors: hypertension, diabetes, smoking, and hyperlipidemia. There are specific 'lacunar syndromes'

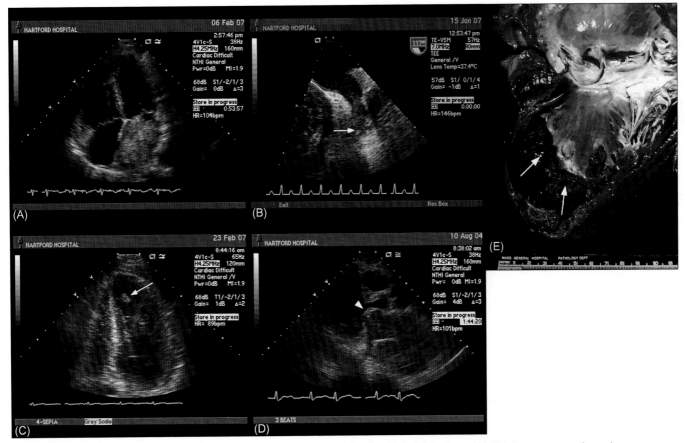

2.2 High-risk cardioembolic sources. Echocardiography shows the following high-risk lesions. (A) Atrial myxoma: an irregular heterogeneous mass involving most of the left atrium, attached to the fossa ovale. (B) Left atrial thrombus in the left atrial appendage (arrow). (C) Thrombus in the thinned apex of the left ventricle following an acute myocardial infarction (arrow). (D) Left atrial thrombus in a patient with rheumatic valvular disease: a parasternal long-axis window shows a 'hockey stick' appearance of the anterior leaflet of the mitral valve (arrowhead). Echocardiography courtesy of Cynthia Taub, MD. (E) Gross pathology shows thrombus within the left ventricle (arrows). Pathology courtesy of Louis Caplan, MD.

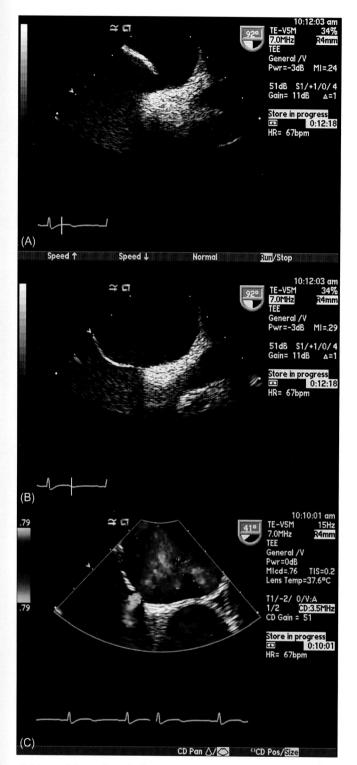

2.3 Low-risk cardioembolic source: patent foramen ovale. A patent foramen ovale is opened (A), closed (B), and with spontaneous left-to-right shunting on color Doppler mode (C) between the left and right atria.

Table 2.2 Cardioembolic causes[7]

High-risk sources
Atrial fibrillation
Rheumatic mitral stenosis
Sick sinus syndrome
Atrial flutter, sustained
Prosthetic valves
Infective endocarditis
Non-bacterial thrombotic endocarditis
Atrial myxoma
Acute myocardial infarction
Aortic atherosclerosis

Low-risk sources
Patent foramen ovale
Atrial septal aneurysm
Mitral valve prolapse
Calcific aortic stenosis and bicuspid aortic sources
Fibroelastomas and Lambl excrescences
Mitral annular calcification

that result from occlusion of these small vessels, including pure motor or pure sensory symptoms, ataxic hemiparesis, dysarthric–clumsy hand syndromes, and simple unilateral sensorimotor deficits, typically presenting without deficits associated with cortical lesions, such as neglect, aphasia, or hemianopia.[11]

The diagnosis of lacunar infarction is made by determining the pattern of deficits on the clinical exam, the history of risk factors and neuroimaging. These small infarcts are best detected initially by diffusion-weighted magnetic resonance imaging (DW-MRI). The acute lesion size of a small vessel infarct is <1.5 cm on T2-weighted MRI sequence and <2.0 cm on DW-MRI sequence (**2.4–2.6**);[12] however, FLAIR (fluid attenuated inversion recovery) MRI sequences are best for grading the severity of chronic small vessel disease (**2.4**).

Other determined etiology

This category refers to less common causes of strokes, such as arterial dissection and other vasculopathies, hypotension, or hypercoagulable states.[13,14] Several of the most common large vessel vasculopathies are surveyed later in this book (Chapter 5).

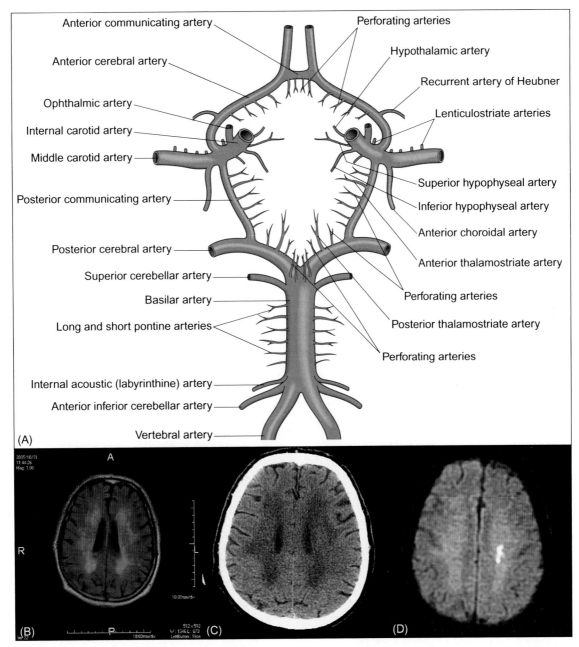

2.4 Small vessel disease. (A) Shows the perforator vessels around the circle of Willis from which most lacunar infarcts arise as a result of arteriolosclerosis. Adapted with permission from Frank Netter, MD. A FLAIR MRI sequence shows severe (B) small vessel disease in the white matter at the level of the lateral ventricles. The CT scan shows this region as a diffuse hypodensity (C), but this modality is not sensitive as a diffusion-weighted MRI sequence (D) in detecting an acute infarct within the chronic small vessel disease.

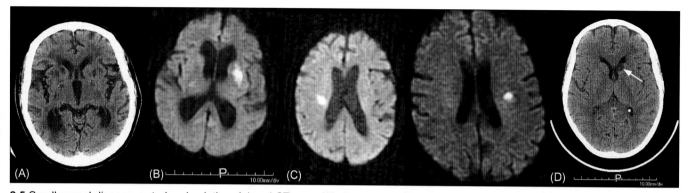

2.5 Small vessel disease, anterior circulation. A head CT scan (A) shows extensive, chronic small vessel lacunar infarcts involving the caudate nucleus and external capsules, bilaterally. An AIS involving left putamen (B) on the diffusion-weighted MRI sequences. Single end-artery strokes in territories of lenticulostriate arteries are seen on diffusion-weighted MRI sequences (C). An old lesion in the head of the left caudate nucleus (arrow) (D).

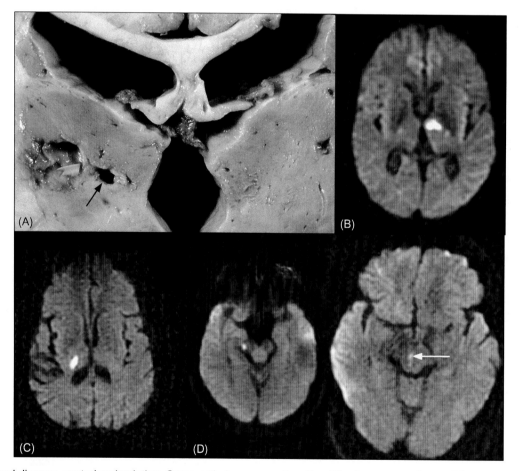

2.6 Small vessel disease, posterior circulation. Gross pathology, coronal section (A), shows a small vessel (thalamostriate) infarct in the thalamus (arrow), adjacent to the third ventricle. Several examples of small vessel strokes seen on diffusion-weighted MRI sequences involving the left medial thalamus (B), the right lateral thalamus (C), the cerebral peduncle (D, left), and the medial midbrain (arrow in D, right image). Pathology courtesy of Robert Schmidt MD, PhD.

Watershed strokes and multifocal peripheral emboli are the most common causes of ischemic strokes that do not localize to a single, specific arterial territory. A differential diagnosis for causes of 'non-arterial' stroke patterns is provided (*Table 2.3*).

Watershed stroke

In cases where a patient becomes hypotensive, a watershed or borderzone infarction can occur. A hemisphere supplied by a stenotic proximal ICA or MCA may be particularly susceptible to low blood pressure due to pump failure, as in cardiac arrhythmia or arrest. However, borderzone infarctions can occur in cases of severe stenosis without hypotension (**case study 1**).

Alternatively, global ischemia due to severe prolonged hypotension may cause bilateral borderzone infarctions even in the absence of proximal stenoses. The low blood pressure usually affects the distal regions of the cerebral hemispheres, with ischemic lesions at borderzone areas between the MCA and anterior cerebral artery (ACA) and the MCA and posterior cerebral artery (PCA), the territory between the superficial and deep penetrating branches of the MCA, and within the cerebellar hemispheres, between the posterior inferior cerebellar artery and superior cerebellar artery distributions (**2.7, 2.8**).[15]

Clinical symptoms of a watershed stroke can include hemiparesis or hemihypesthesia with predominance in the leg or proximal arm, depending on involvement of the motor and/or sensory cortex. When the infarction is bilateral, proximal weakness of all four extremities, the so-called 'man-in-the-barrel' syndrome, may result, along with cognitive impairment.[16] Patients suffering bilateral watershed infarctions have overall poorer outcomes than patients with strokes in most other distributions.[17]

When hypoperfusion is severe, such as during a prolonged cardiac arrest, a syndrome of global anoxic–ischemic encephalopathy results, with diffuse cerebral edema associated with high mortality (**2.9**).

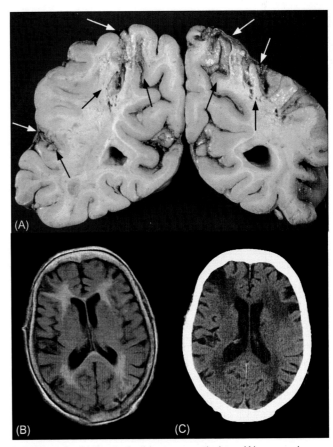

2.7 Watershed infarcts. In this gross pathology (A), coronal section, note encephalomalacia and loss of normal gyral architecture in the parieto-occipital region bilaterally (arrows), a borderzone between the MCA and PCA territories. A FLAIR MRI sequence (B) and matching head CT scan (C) show typical bihemispheric (ACA–MCA and MCA–PCA) borderzone infarcts. Pathology courtesy of Robert Schmidt MD, PhD.

Table 2.3 Stroke etiologies with non-arterial distributions

- Watershed lesions
- Multifocal emboli
- Venous infarction*
- Vasculitis*
- Degenerative vasculopathies, e.g., moyamoya disease, sickle cell disease
- Reversible posterior leukoencephalopathy syndrome
- Metabolic etiologies, e.g., mitochondrial disease (mitochondrial myopathy, encephalopathy, lactic acidosis, and stroke or MELAS)
- Leukoencephalopathies, e.g., CADASIL
- Non-vascular lesions, e.g., metastatic disease*

*Often associated with a hemorrhagic component.

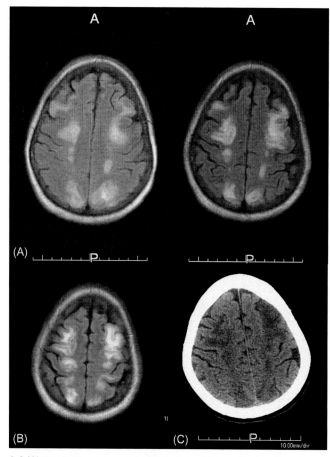

2.8 Watershed versus embolic lesions. This patient suffered cardiogenic shock prior to cardiac valvular replacement. The lesions on the FLAIR MRI (A,B) and CT scan (C) suggest an embolic pattern at lower levels (A) but have a more confluent pattern at higher levels (B,C) consistent with a watershed pattern.

Multifocal emboli

Small, multifocal emboli typically migrate to distal, borderzone territories (**2.10**). Watershed and embolic strokes may often coexist (**2.8**). A low-flow state, most commonly caused by pump (cardiac) failure, may contribute to the poor 'washout' of microemboli. Patients in the cardiovascular ICU with stroke often have a pattern consistent with both diffuse multifocal emboli and borderzone lesions.[18]

Undetermined etiology

Even after exhaustive diagnostic studies, a certain number of strokes will have an undetermined cause, a percentage as high as 30% in some studies.[19] This category also includes

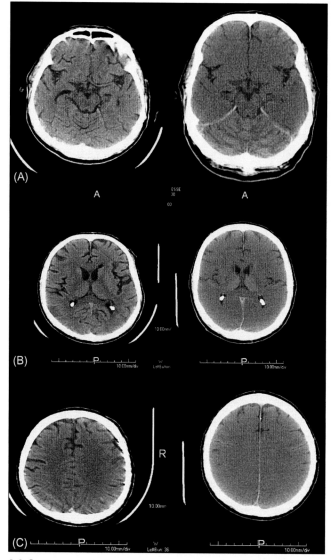

2.9 Severe anoxic–ischemic encephalopathy. This patient suffered two cardiac arrests, and had CT scans after each one. The first scan (left panels) is juxtaposed with the second (right panels), at several levels: midbrain (A), choroid plexus calcifications (B), and cerebral hemispheres above the lateral ventricles (C). Before the second CT scan, a more protracted arrest caused diffuse, severe cerebral edema seen in the complete effacement of the sulci in the second study (right panels).

patients who have more than one feasible stroke etiology. For example, a young woman with a history of tobacco use and complicated migraine, who presents with a stroke and a diagnostic work-up positive for a lower extremity deep vein thrombosis and a patent foramen ovale, has multiple possible contributing etiologies.

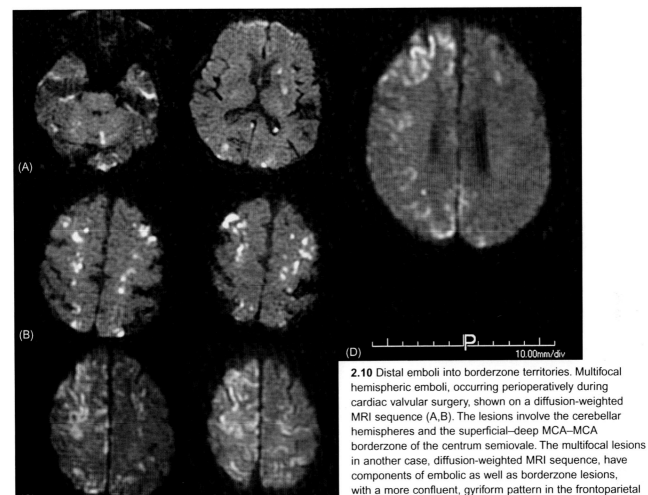

2.10 Distal emboli into borderzone territories. Multifocal hemispheric emboli, occurring perioperatively during cardiac valvular surgery, shown on a diffusion-weighted MRI sequence (A,B). The lesions involve the cerebellar hemispheres and the superficial–deep MCA–MCA borderzone of the centrum semiovale. The multifocal lesions in another case, diffusion-weighted MRI sequence, have components of embolic as well as borderzone lesions, with a more confluent, gyriform pattern in the frontoparietal region (C,D).

Case studies

Case study 1. Large vessel disease: intracranial stenosis causing borderzone infarctions

A 59-year-old woman with a history of tobacco use presents with fluctuating right hemibody symptoms (fluctuating right arm and leg weakness and paresthesias), and was found to have watershed (borderzone) ischemic lesions on diffusion-weighted MRI (DW-MRI) sequence (**CS 1.1**A), with low perfusion on the cerebral blood flow map (CT perfusion, **CS 1.1**B).

The etiology was identified as severe left distal M1/proximal M2 stenosis without hypotension, difficult to visualize on a coronal cervical and intracranial MRA study (**CS 1.2**A) but magnified on CT angiography (arrow) (**CS 1.2**B). Angioplasty was performed with a 2-mm

Maverick balloon, immediately before deployment of a 3×9-mm Wingspan™ stent. A post-procedural non-contrast CT scan shows the stent as a hyperdense region coursing into the Sylvian fissure (**CS 1.2**C).

A second patient with borderzone infarction had a comparable lesion, a right mid-M1 stenosis (**CS 1.3**) shown

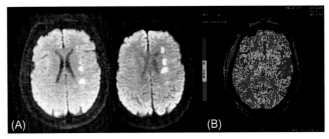

CS 1.1

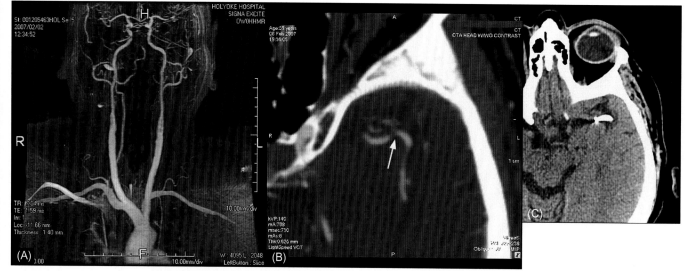

CS 1.2

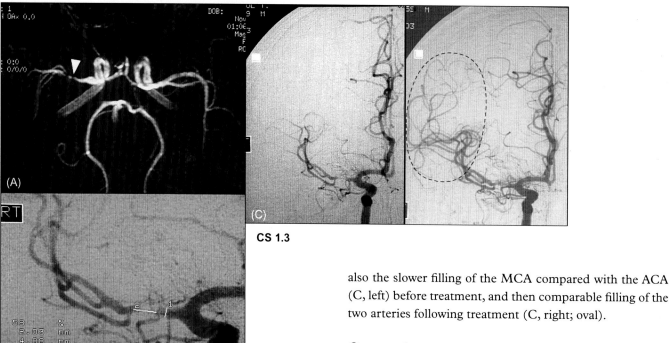

CS 1.3

first on MRA (arrowhead) (A). Conventional angiography, (B, C) demonstrates near-occlusive intracranial MCA disease. Elective angioplasty was performed; the lesion is first measured (B); the true lumen of the MCA is >2.0 mm, and the lesion is nearly 5 mm long. Pre-angioplasty (C, left) versus post-angioplasty (C, right) angiography shows improved vessel diameter of the stenotic region. Notice also the slower filling of the MCA compared with the ACA (C, left) before treatment, and then comparable filling of the two arteries following treatment (C, right; oval).

Comments

Endovascular technology is evolving to transform the management of large vessel intracranial and extracranial disease. Although the experience with angioplasty and stenting for extracranial ICA atherostenosis is extensive, with many randomized clinical trials published,[21] clear guidelines are not established for the management of intracranial disease. Some early periprocedural data for the Gateway balloon-Wingspan™ stent system in patients with symptomatic intracranial disease found a high rate of technical success and acceptable periprocedural morbidity.[22]

These techniques may be useful for elective, secondary prevention as well as emergency revascularization. The risks of endovascular cervical and intracranial procedures include reperfusion injury (e.g., the carotid reperfusion syndrome); perforator infarction; arterial dissection; and distal emboli.[23]

Case study 2. Cardioembolic disease: calcific embolism causing middle cerebral artery stroke

History

A 36-year-old man developed a left hemispheric stroke syndrome during a cardiac catheterization procedure. He had a history of a congenital bicuspid aortic valve, and was undergoing catheterization to assess his risk for coronary heart disease and the status of his aortic stenosis. Given femoral access already in place from the cardiac procedure, a distal left ICA occlusion was identified on fluoroscopy, where intra-arterial tissue plasminogen activator, 25 mg, was infused prior to transfer to the regional stroke center.

Clinical course

Hospital day (HD) 1

On arrival, the patient was taken directly to the interventional neuroradiology suite. Conventional angiography, anteroposterior view, left ICA injection (**CS 2.1**) shows occlusion of the M1 segment (arrowhead) (A, left). After recanalization efforts using a clot retrieval device, the Mechanical Embolus Removal in Cerebral Ischemia (MERCI) LX, and angioplasty in the first- and second-order MCA (M1 and M2) segments, multiple filling defects are still observed within both the left first-order ACA (A1) and M1 segments (A, right). On a lateral view (B), the guidewire is shown entering the M1 segment, with excellent flow into the A1 (arrow) and A2 (arrowheads) segments (left). With the guidewire removed, flow into the M1 segment remains quite limited, with heterogeneous flow within the distal ICA (arrowhead) and proximal ACA and MCA branches (right). During this procedure, the interventional neuroradiologist noted a large occlusive piece of particulate matter, >2 mm, shifting between the M1 and A1 segments around the distal ICA.

HD 2–3

*   *MCA occlusion* (**CS 2.2**): A calcified 'hyper-hyperdense' MCA sign is shown on the non-contrast head CT scan (A,B), and on MRI (C), as a hypointense signal (arrow) on the source images of the intracranial MR angiogram at

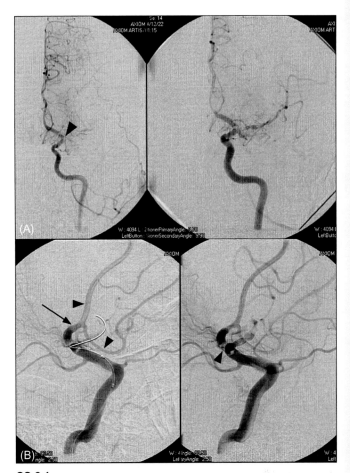

CS 2.1

the level of the circle of Willis (C, left), and no flow registers into the left M1 segment on the MRA (C, right).

*   *Transesophageal echocardiography* (**CS 2.3**): The source of the MCA lesion is confirmed on a long axis view of the aortic valve demonstrating the presence of valvular thickening and calcification (A), and a short axis view of the aortic valve during systole (B).

Follow-up CT scans (**CS 2.4**) on HD4 (A) and at 6 months post-stroke (B) document the large left MCA stroke.

Comments

Stroke in the setting of cardiac catheterization is not uncommon, and is attributed to the dislodgement of clot or atheromatous debris off the aortic arch or directly from the guide catheter tip, and less frequently, valvular debris.[24] In this case, the initial head CT scan and echocardiography identified the stroke etiology as particulate thromboembolism emanating from the patient's calcified aortic valve.

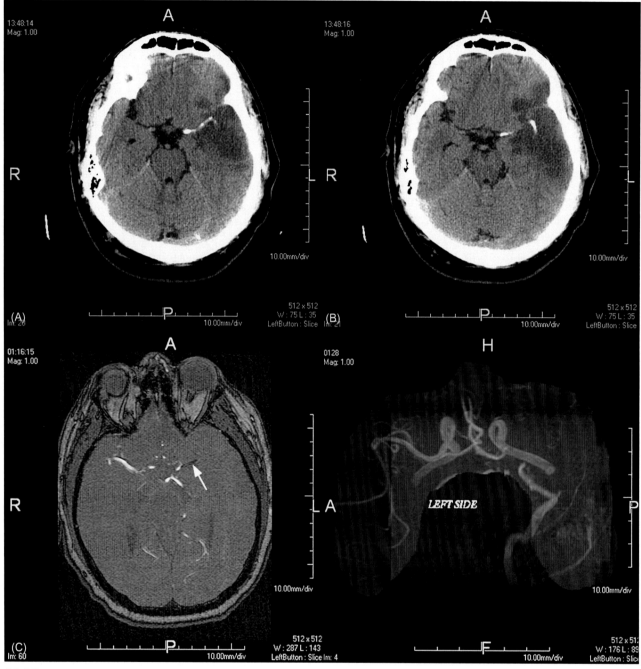

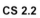
CS 2.2

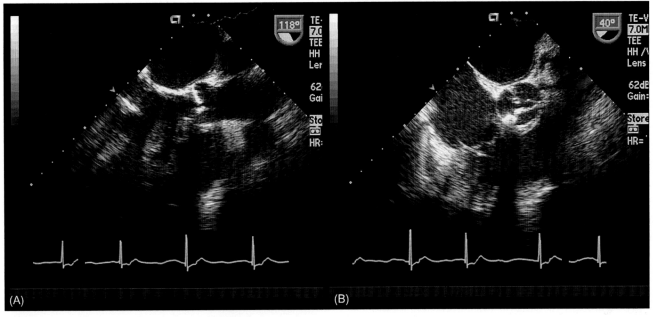

CS 2.3

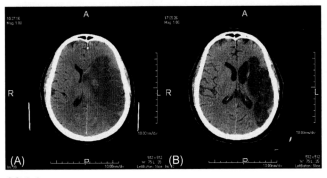

CS 2.4

References

1. Adams H, Jr, Bendixen B, Kappelle L, *et al.* Classification of acute ischemic stroke: definition for use in a multicenter trial. *Stroke* 1993; **24**: 35–41.

2. Publications Committee for the Trial of ORG 10172 in Acute Stroke Treatment (TOAST) Investigators. Low molecular weight heparinoid, ORG 10172 (Danaparoid) and outcome after acute ischemic stroke: a randomized controlled trial. *JAMA* 1998; **279**: 1265–72.

3. Selwa L, Chimowitz M. Atherosclerotic intracranial large artery occlusive disease. *Neurologist* 1995; **1**: 53–64.

4. Amarenco P, Cohen A, Tzourio C, *et al.* Atherosclerotic disease of the aortic arch and the risk of ischemic stroke. *N Engl J Med* 1994; **331**: 1474–9.

5. French Study of Aortic Plaques in Stroke Group. Atherosclerotic disease of the aortic arch as a risk factor for recurrent ischemic stroke. *N Engl J Med* 1996; **334**: 1216–21.

6. Ezekowitz M, Levine J. Preventing stroke in patients with atrial fibrillation. *JAMA* 1999; **281**: 1830–5.

7. Schneck MJ, Xu L, Palacio S. Cardioembolic Stroke 2005. (Accessed at http://www.emedicine.com/neuro/topic45.htm/ from eMedicine, last updated February 13, 2008).

8. Mas J-L, Arquizan C, Lamy C, *et al.* Recurrent cerebrovascular events associated with patent foramen ovale, atrial septal aneurysm, or both. *N Engl J Med* 2001; **345**: 1740–6.

9. Rahmatullah A, Rahko P, Stein J. Transesophageal echocardiography for the evaluation and management of patients with cerebral ischemia. *Clin Cardiol* 1999; **22**: 391–6.

10. Albers G, Amarenco P, Easton J, Sacco R, Teal P. Antithrombotic and thrombolytic therapy for ischemic stroke: The Seventh ACCP Conference on Antithrombotic and Thrombolytic Therapy. *Chest* 2004; **3**: S483–512.

11. Fisher C. Lacunar infarcts: a review. *Cerebrovasc Dis* 1991; **1**: 311–20.

12. Wessels T, Rottger C, Jauss M, Kaps M, Traupe H, Stolz E. Identification of embolic stroke patterns by

diffusion-weighted MRI in clinically defined lacunar stroke syndromes. *Stroke* 2005; **36**: 757–61.

13. Blecic S, Bogousslavsky J. Other uncommon angiopathies. In: Bogousslavsky J, Caplan L, eds. *Uncommon Causes of Stroke*. New York: Cambridge University Press; 2001: 355–68.

14. Bogousslavsky J, Caplan L. *Uncommon Causes of Stroke*. New York: Cambridge University Press; 2001.

15. Kumral E, Ozdemirkiran T, Alper Y. Strokes in the subinsular territory: clinical, topographical, and etiological patterns. *Neurology* 2004; **63**: 2429–32.

16. Bogousslavsky J, Hommel M. Ischemic stroke syndromes: clinical features, anatomy, vascular territories. In: Adams H, Jr, ed. *Handbook of Cerebrovascular Diseases*. New York: Marcel Dekker; 1993: 51–94.

17. Gottesman R, Sherman P, Grega M, *et al.* Watershed strokes after cardiac surgery. *Stroke* 2006; **37**: 2306–11.

18. Caplan L, Hennerici M. Impaired clearance of emboli (washout) is an important link between hypoperfusion, embolism, and ischemic stroke. *Arch Neurol* 1998; **55**: 1475–82.

19. Foulkes M, Wolf P, Price T, Morh J, Hier D. The Stroke Data Bank: design, methods, and baseline characteristics. *Stroke* 1988; **19**: 547–54.

20. Osborn A. The aortic arch and great vessels. In: *Diagnostic Cerebral Angiography*, 2nd edn. Philadelphia: Lippincott Williams & Wilkins; 1999: 1–29.

21. Furlan A. Carotid-artery stenting — case open or closed? [editorial]. *N Engl J Med* 2006; **355**: 1726–9.

22. Fiorella D, Levy E, Turk A, *et al.* US multicenter experience with the Wingspan stent system for the treatment of intracranial atheromatous disease: periprocedural results. *Stroke* 2007; **38**: 881–7.

23. Levy E, Chaturvedi S. Perforator stroke following intracranial stenting: a sacrifice for the greater good? *Neurology* 2006; **66**: 1803–4.

24. Khatri P, Kasner S. Ischemic strokes after cardiac catheterization: opportune thrombolysis candidates? *Arch Neurol* 2006; **63**: 817–21.

Further reading

Adams H, Jr, Bendixen B, Kappelle L, *et al.* Classification of acute ischemic stroke: definition for use in a multicenter trial. *Stroke* 1993; **24**: 35–41.

Bogousslavsky J, Caplan L. *Stroke Syndromes*, 2nd edn. New York: Cambridge University Press; 2001.

Chapter 3

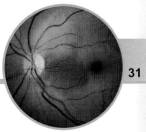

Anterior Circulation

Introduction: anatomy

The arterial site of an embolic or thrombotic occlusion determines the anatomic classification of an ischemic stroke. Strokes within the distribution of the carotid arteries are referred to as lesions of the anterior circulation, and strokes within the distribution of the vertebrobasilar arteries are referred to as lesions of the posterior circulation.

The major arteries of the anterior circulation are the internal carotid (ICA), middle cerebrals (MCA), and anterior cerebrals (ACA). Eighty percent of blood flow to the brain runs through the carotid system. The major arteries of the posterior circulation are the vertebrals, basilar, and the posterior cerebrals (PCA) (3.1A,B). Neuroimaging studies, either computed tomography (CT) or magnetic resonance imaging (MRI) scans, can identify the arterial territory and size of acute infarcts. Outstanding MRI-based mappings of the anterior and posterior arterial circulations have been published (e.g., 3.1C).[1,2]

A critical predictor of stroke outcomes is the competency of the collateral circulation to arteries adjacent to the occluded vessel. The primary anastomoses exist through the circle of Willis, connecting the major arteries of the anterior and posterior circulation systems via the anterior and posterior communicating arteries (3.2A; case study 1).[3] This circle is complete in approximately 25% of normal individuals. There are also important secondary collateral pathways provided by leptomeningeal vessels linking the territories of the MCA and the ACA and the MCA and the PCA (3.2B).[4] During a proximal MCA occlusion, retrograde collateral flow can be supplied from the adjacent ACA leptomeningeal segments that supply the peripheral MCA territory (3.2C,D).

Internal carotid artery territory

Proximal internal carotid artery

The most common site for large vessel atherosclerosis (TOAST mechanism 1) is at the carotid bifurcation (3.3–3.6).[5] Other typical locations are in the carotid siphon and the proximal common carotid artery. Most often, symptomatic carotid atherosclerotic disease results in artery-to-artery embolism to its MCA territory (3.6). Occlusion of the ICA can result in a wide range of lesions, from multifocal small embolic ischemic lesions (3.6A,B) to massive hemispheric stroke (3.7).[6,7]

Intracranial branches

The ICA has seven segments named for adjacent structures (3.3A). There are no extracranial branches, but typically there are three intracranial branches proximal to the terminal bifurcation of the ICA into the MCA and ACA.[8,9] These branches are the ophthalmic artery, the posterior communicating artery, and the anterior choroidal artery (3.8). The ophthalmic artery chiefly supplies the eye, via its branching into an end-artery, the central retinal artery.[10] An embolism to the central retinal artery commonly results in monocular blindness due to infarction of the retina (3.9). Embolism to the anterior choroidal artery is rare (3.10).[11]

Distal internal carotid artery branches

The ICA terminates with its division into the MCA and ACA. This is called the 'carotid T' because of its appearance (3.11A,B). An occlusion of the ICA terminus, a carotid T lesion, is a common cause of severe stroke (3.7, 3.11, 3.12). The thrombus occludes the distal-most part of the ICA, extending into the proximal segments of the MCA (M1)

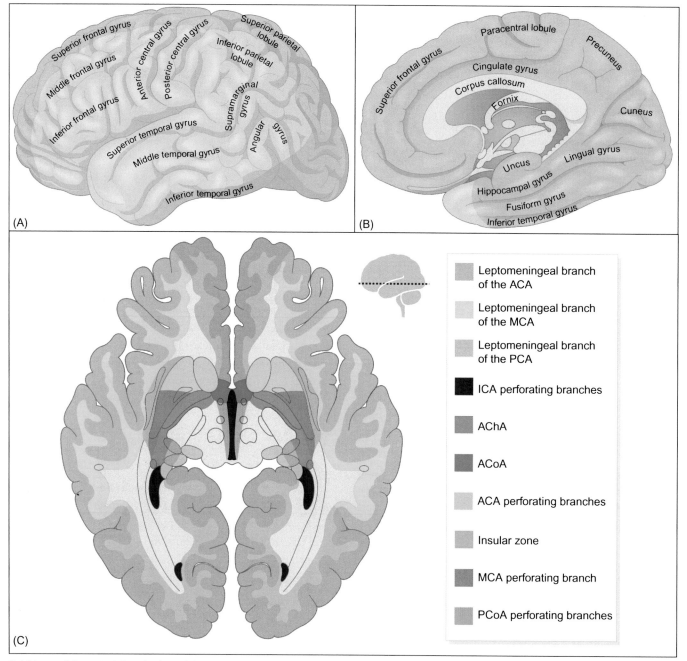

3.1 Maps of the arterial territories of the cerebral hemispheres. Lateral (A) and medial (B) views of the ACA, MCA, and PCA territories indicated by the following colors: orange, blue and pink, respectively. A MRI-based mapping of major artery territories at a lower level of the cerebral hemispheres, with its associated color-guided arterial key. AChA, anterior choroidal artery; ACoA, anterior communicating artery; ICA, internal carotid artery; PCoA, posterior communicating artery. Redrawn with permission, from Tatu *et al.*[2]

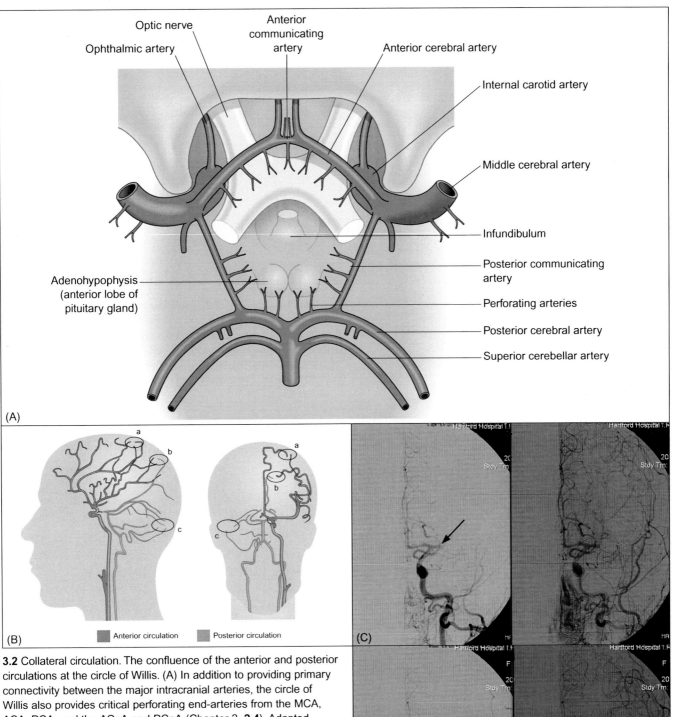

3.2 Collateral circulation. The confluence of the anterior and posterior circulations at the circle of Willis. (A) In addition to providing primary connectivity between the major intracranial arteries, the circle of Willis also provides critical perforating end-arteries from the MCA, ACA, PCA, and the ACoA and PCoA (Chapter 2, **2.4**). Adapted from Osborn.[3] Intracranial arterial collateral circulation systems are shown in lateral and frontal views (B). Common secondary pathways are the leptomeningeal anastomoses between the ACA and MCA (a), and between the PCA and MCA (b); as well as tectal plexus between PCA and SCA (c). Adapted from Liebeskind.[4] A conventional angiogram (anteroposterior view) of a left M1 occlusion (arrow) (C, left). A later phase image shows some ACA and leptomeningeal collateral flow over the left hemisphere (C, right). Following recanalization of the M1 occlusion (D), note the balanced ACA and MCA flow in early (D, left) and later (D, right) stages of dye injection.

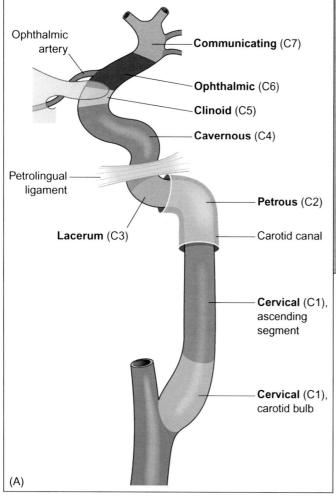

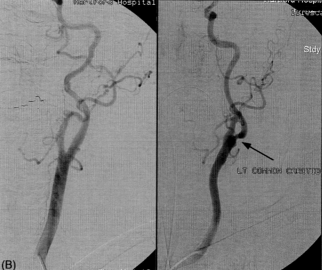

3.3 ICA and carotid bifurcation. The course and branches of the cervical and intracranial ICA, with its segments, named for adjacent structures: the cervical, petrous, lacerum, cavernous, clinoid, ophthalmic, and communicating segments (A). Adapted with permission from Osborn.[8,9] Two conventional angiographic images of the carotid bifurcation (B). The first study (left) shows only mild atherosclerosis, while the second (right) shows typical proximal ICA plaque (arrow). Extensive branching of the external carotid arteries is seen, while the internal carotid artery has no cervical branches.

and ACA (A1). Rarely, the entire cerebral hemisphere may be at risk, either because the ICA territory also includes the PCA territory due to a fetal PCA circulation (Chapter 4, **4.17**), or because rapid uncal herniation creates an occlusive mass effect on the ipsilateral PCA (**3.12**).

Symptoms of internal carotid artery stroke

When the ICA is occluded, the clinical syndrome is usually one of an MCA occlusion. The anterior communicating artery typically prevents infarction of the ipsilateral ACA by preserving blood flow from the contralateral ICA. The next two sections review symptomatology of MCA and ACA infarcts.

Middle cerebral artery territory

The initial segment of the MCA, known as the M1 or first-order division, is a direct continuation of the distal ICA and is larger than its adjacent counterpart in the ACA, the A1 segment (**3.13; case study 1**). Thromboembolic material in the anterior circulation tends to flow into the distribution of the MCA, making it by far the most common territory for ischemic stroke. Strokes within an MCA territory may also be subdivided by the location of the occlusion within the MCA, more proximal M1 and M2 lesions (first- and second-order divisions) versus more distal M3 and M4 lesions (opercular and cortical branches, respectively) (**3.13–3.19**).[12]

Text continued on page 42

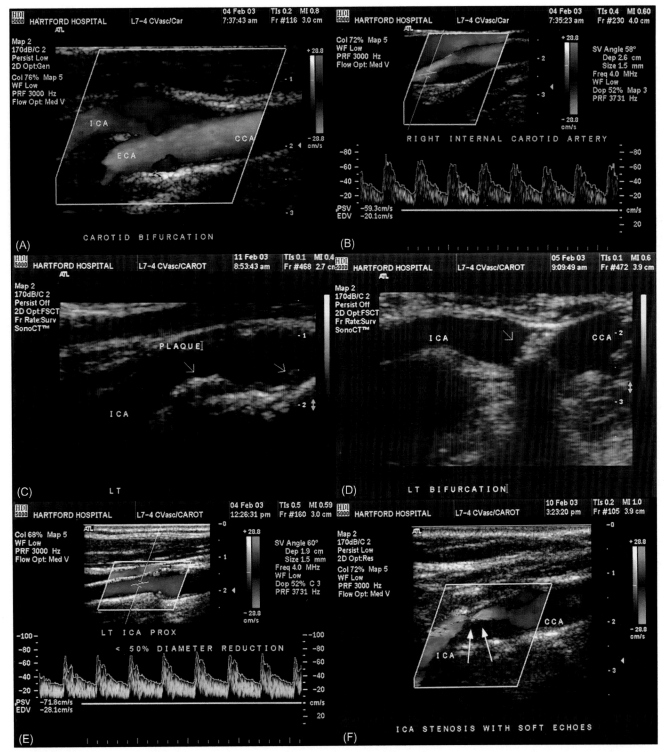

3.4 Normal and abnormal carotid anatomy, Doppler sonography. Normal carotid bifurcation, color Doppler (A). Normal waveform with peak systolic velocity of 70 cm/s and end diastolic velocity of 25 cm/s is shown (B). Two areas of smooth echogenic plaque are identified by arrows (C). Calcified plaque creates a bright echogenic region that causes shadowing (arrow) (D). Carotid stenosis <50% causes minimal change in the baseline velocities (E). This area of smooth plaque (arrows) caused 80–99% stenosis, calculated by marked velocity elevations (peak systolic velocity of 605 cm/s and end diastolic velocity of 211 cm/s) (F). Images courtesy of Janice Guica, RN, RVT.

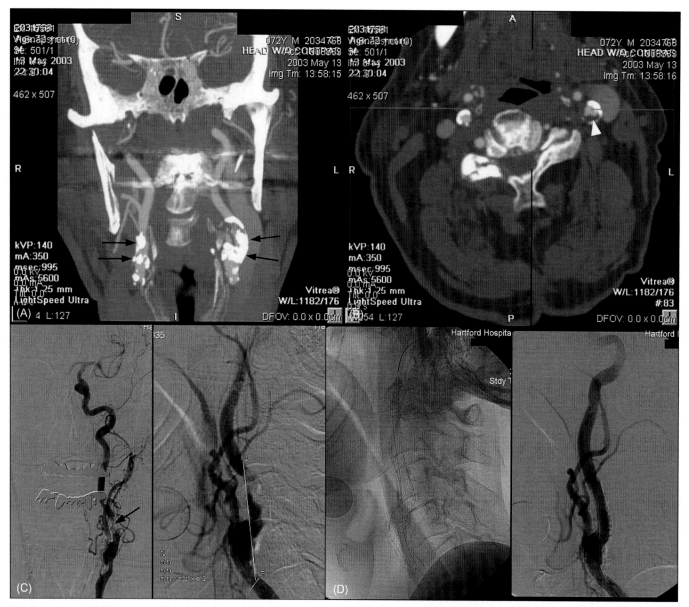

3.5 Severe carotid atherosclerotic disease. CT angiography, coronal image (A), documents heavy calcified carotid bifurcations, bilaterally; the hyperdense patches are calcified plaque (arrows). Transaxial cuts of the CT angiogram above the level of the carotid bifurcation shows the proximal ICA and ECA, documenting calcium, thrombus (arrowhead), and reduced true lumen in the left ICA (B). Conventional angiography, left common carotid artery injection, documents a high-grade stenosis above the bifurcation of the ICA (arrow) (C, left), an area magnified and measured for angioplasty and stenting (C, right). Following the placement of two stents, before (D, left) and during (D, right) carotid injection, demonstrating excellent flow through the formerly near-occlusive lesion on the latter image.

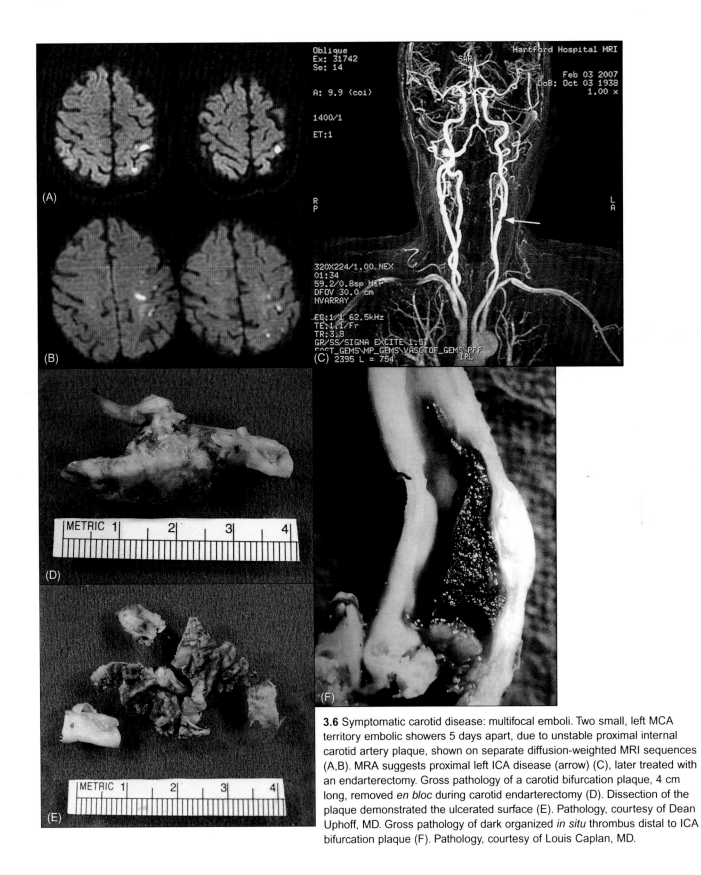

3.6 Symptomatic carotid disease: multifocal emboli. Two small, left MCA territory embolic showers 5 days apart, due to unstable proximal internal carotid artery plaque, shown on separate diffusion-weighted MRI sequences (A,B). MRA suggests proximal left ICA disease (arrow) (C), later treated with an endarterectomy. Gross pathology of a carotid bifurcation plaque, 4 cm long, removed *en bloc* during carotid endarterectomy (D). Dissection of the plaque demonstrated the ulcerated surface (E). Pathology, courtesy of Dean Uphoff, MD. Gross pathology of dark organized *in situ* thrombus distal to ICA bifurcation plaque (F). Pathology, courtesy of Louis Caplan, MD.

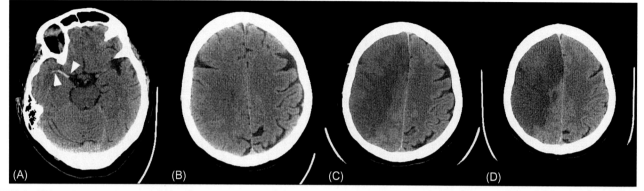

3.7 Right ICA territory stroke in evolution. Non-contrasted CT scan demonstrates a hyperdense distal ICA/proximal MCA sign (arrowheads) signifying acute thrombus involving these arteries (A). The following three images show the progressively demarcated infarction in the right ACA and MCA territories, on admission, with loss of sulcal markings consistent with early edema (B), 1 day later (C), and 2 days later (D).

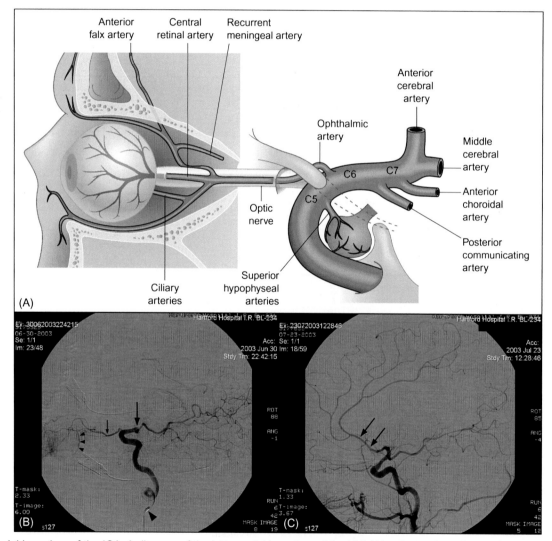

3.8 Intracranial branches of the ICA. A diagram of the intracranial branches of the ICA (A); adapted from Osborn.[8] Two angiographic studies, lateral images, of carotid injections. (B) Distal ICA (carotid T) lesion, just distal to the PCoA (arrow), with most choroidal flow appreciated via the posterior choroidal artery. The distal catheter tip is shown (arrowhead), as is the ophthalmic artery (small arrow) and the choroidal blush of the eye (small arrowheads); (C) Distal ICA/proximal MCA (M1) occlusion. The lack of visualization of the MCA, occluded proximally, enables an excellent view of the entire ACA (arrows are on A2 segment).

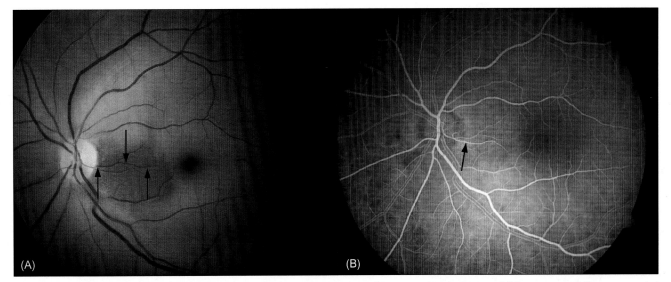

3.9 Retinal stroke. Acute-onset painless vision loss occurs with occlusion of the central retinal artery. Vision was partially recovered due to maintenance of macular blood supply via a patent cilioretinal artery (arrows), shown here on fundus photograph (A) and fluorescein angiography (B).

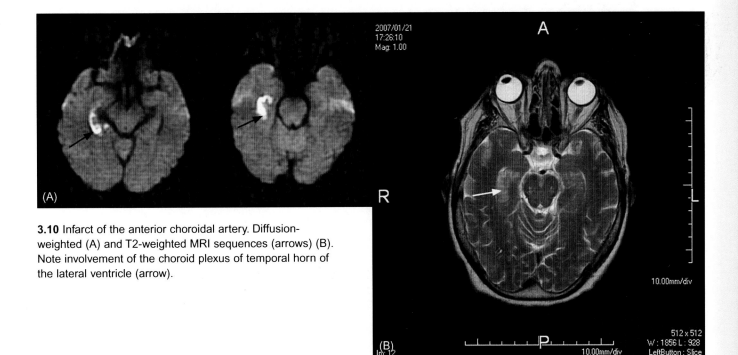

3.10 Infarct of the anterior choroidal artery. Diffusion-weighted (A) and T2-weighted MRI sequences (arrows) (B). Note involvement of the choroid plexus of temporal horn of the lateral ventricle (arrow).

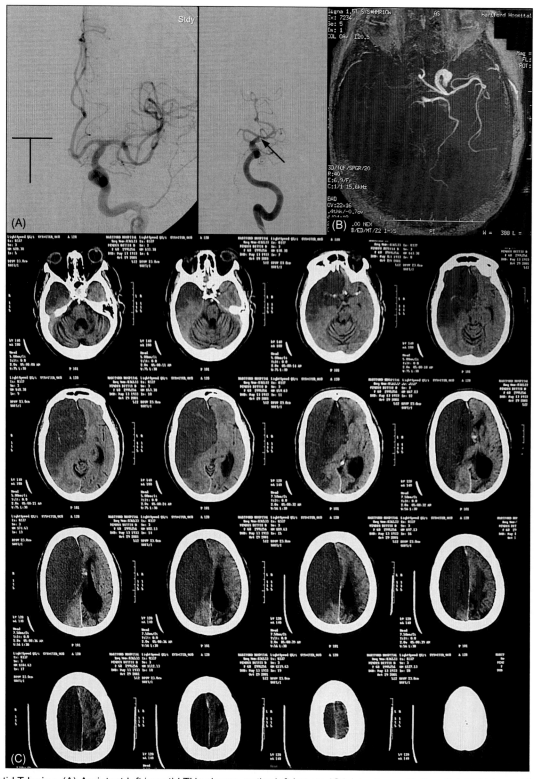

3.11 The carotid T lesion. (A) An intact left 'carotid T' is shown on the left image, ICA injection, with the distal ICA branching into the ACA (medial branch) and MCA (lateral branch). A carotid T occlusion is shown on the right. A sharp cut-off of the artery is marked (arrow), with no flow into the ACA or MCA. Most of the flow is seen posteriorly into the adjacent PCA territory. A composite transaxial (top-down) view, intracranial MRA (B) shows almost no signal in the right intracranial ICA, in contrast to the normal left side. A right ICA-distribution stroke on composite CT images (C): note the midline mass effect, squeezing the midbrain and trapping the contralateral lateral ventricle.

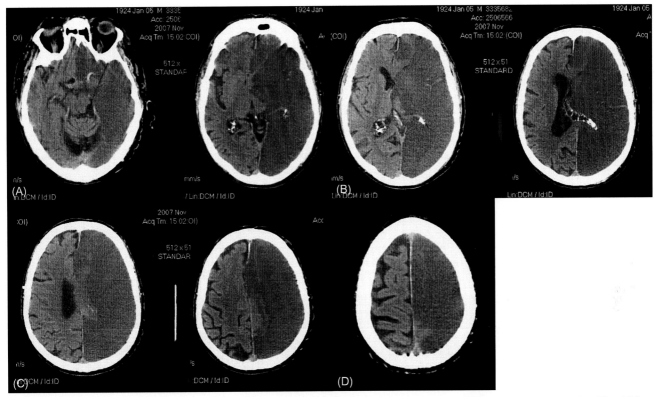

3.12 Stroke of the entire left hemisphere due to ICA occlusion. The infarct involves the ACA, MCA, and PCA territories. The ACA territory has infarcted because there is no ACoA and/or due to subfalcine herniation. The PCA territory has infarcted because of mass effect caused by uncal herniation. Note the spared left-sided territories: midbrain, medial thalamus, rostrum of the corpus callosum, and some parasagittal cortex.

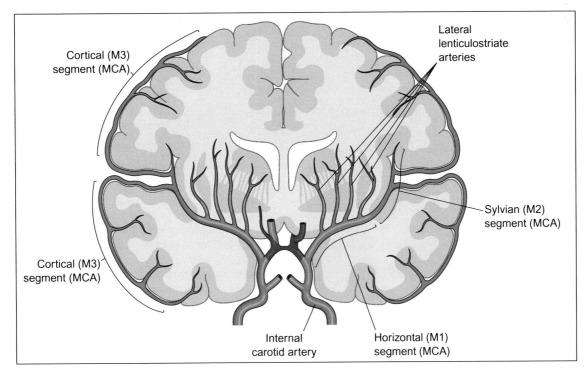

3.13 Anatomy of the MCA. A coronal illustration of the proximal MCA and lenticulostriate perforating arteries around the circle of Willis, as well as the more distal divisions of the MCA.

M1 occlusion

M1 occlusions may occur proximal to the lenticulostriate perforating arteries, blocking flow to cortical and subcortical structures. The lenticulostriate arteries supply the internal capsule and other adjacent subcortical structures and are end-arteries (without collateral circulation). The malignant MCA syndrome, in which significant hemispheric edema develops, carries a 70–80% mortality rate with medical treatment only (**3.14**).[13] Uncommonly, downward herniation may also occlude the ipsilateral PCA, resulting in infarction of medial temporal and occipital lobes (**3.15**).

Perforating branches

Occlusion of the lenticulostriate small vessels is the most common site for lacunar stroke syndromes. The medial lenticulostriates (from the proximal MCA near the ICA bifurcation) and the lateral lenticulostriates (from the distal half of the M1 segment) are the largest group of small intracranial perforator vessels. Lacunar syndromes in this region usually affect the basal ganglia, internal capsule, caudate nucleus, lentiform nucleus, as well as the periventricular white-matter (e.g., Chapter 2, **2.4**, **2.5**). Lacunar strokes can result from intrinsic disease of the perforating artery (TOAST mechanism 3) or from occlusion of the MCA supplying the perforating arteries. Larger branch-artery occlusive disease such as partial occlusion of the M1 segment may result in larger, confluent subcortical lesions, colloquially known as 'lagunes' (i.e., for giant lacunes) or 'macunes' (i.e., for major lacunes) (**3.16**).[14]

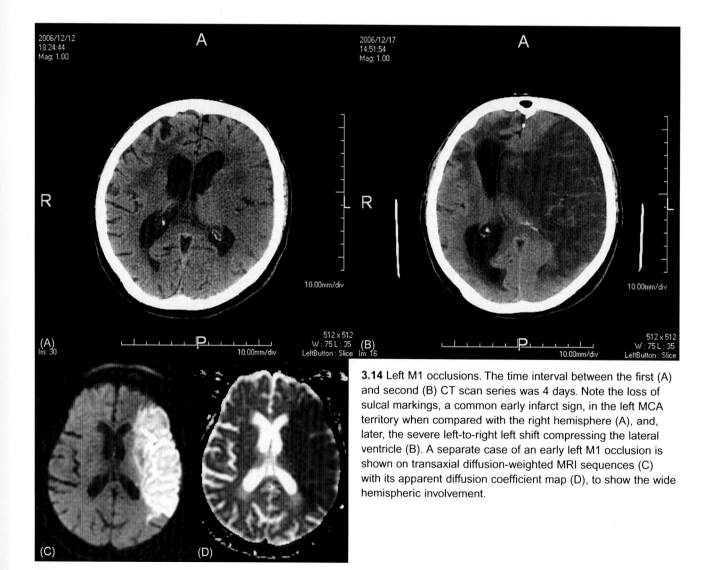

3.14 Left M1 occlusions. The time interval between the first (A) and second (B) CT scan series was 4 days. Note the loss of sulcal markings, a common early infarct sign, in the left MCA territory when compared with the right hemisphere (A), and, later, the severe left-to-right left shift compressing the lateral ventricle (B). A separate case of an early left M1 occlusion is shown on transaxial diffusion-weighted MRI sequences (C) with its apparent diffusion coefficient map (D), to show the wide hemispheric involvement.

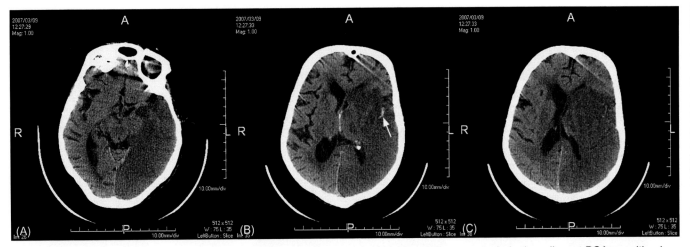

3.15 MCA plus PCA infarction. An acute MCA occlusion causing supratentorial herniation may occlude the adjacent PCA, resulting in a combined MCA/PCA infarction. Note the mass effect on the midbrain (A), involvement of lenticulostriate areas and the head of the caudate nucleus (B,C), and an area of hemorrhagic transformation (arrow) (B). (An alternative mechanism is embolism from an ICA atherosclerotic disease into both a fetal PCA and an adjacent MCA).

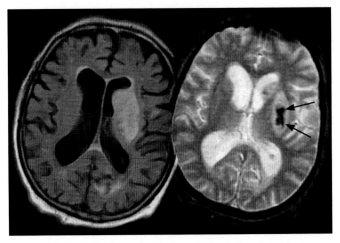

3.16 A 'Macune.' A subcortical infarct in the left periventricular white matter on MRI sequences: a FLAIR (left), and the gradient echo (GE) sequence (right) demonstrates hemorrhagic transformation (arrows) of this lesion.

Cortical branches

M2 occlusions occur distal to the lenticulostriate arteries and will usually produce predominantly cortical infarction. These lesions may be quite large, and a practical clinical differentiation is between the superior and inferior division M2 lesions described in the next section on symptoms (**3.17**, **3.18**).

M3 and M4 occlusions occur in one or two of the distal-most branches of the MCA. The area of infarction and symptoms will depend on which individual branch is occluded. Each M2 or M3 segment (stem artery) gives rise to one to five cortical M4 branches, for a total of 12 major cortical areas (**3.19**).[12] Individual M4 branch infarctions are typically the result of occlusion by small emboli (**3.20**) or may result after resolution of a more proximal M2 or M3 occlusion (**3.21**).

Multifocal embolic showers are quite common sequelae of atheroembolism from more proximal sources. Aortic and cardiac sources (TOAST mechanisms 1 and 2) have the potential to cause bilateral hemispheric infarcts, and emboli from the carotid bifurcation (TOAST mechanism 1) may cause multiple ipsilateral hemispheric infarcts (**3.6**, **3.20**, **3.21**). Small cholesterol-laden emboli from the ICA and emboli from other sources, such as intracardiac thrombus, carotid dissection, or bacterial endocarditis, may also cause distal occlusions.

As MCA occlusion is the most common location for infarction, high-risk patients may suffer recurrent strokes in the same territory. Both CT and MRI scans can document sequential lesions, to offer a record of acute-upon-chronic strokes (**3.22**).

Neuroimaging can track the progression of an acute infarct, predicting the eventual lesion size (**3.23**).

Symptoms of middle cerebral artery stroke[6,12,15]

Stroke symptoms depend on which section of the MCA is occluded, whether there is total or partial (branch) occlusion, the pathophysiology (large vessel versus small vessel disease), and the laterality of the lesion (right versus left hemisphere).

Text continued on page 48

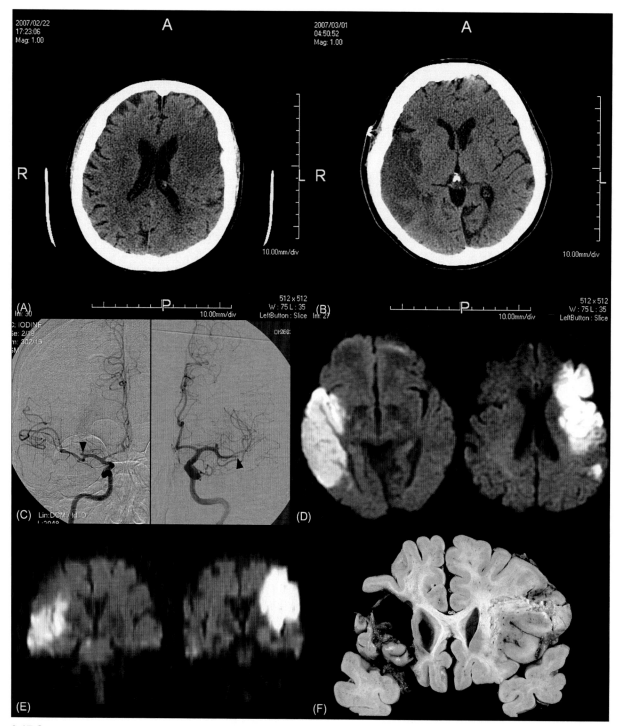

3.17 Superior versus inferior M2 territory lesions. Occlusions of the M2 superior and inferior divisions of the MCA are juxtaposed, beyond or at the level of the MCA bifurcation, on early CT scans, A (superior), B (inferior). Angiography of ICA injections, showing a superior M2 branch acute occlusion (C, left) and an inferior M2-branch (C, right) (arrowheads). An inferior M2 division stroke (left) and a superior M2 division stroke (right) shown on transaxial diffusion-weighted MRI sequences (D); and reconstructed coronal diffusion-weighted MRI (E). Gross pathology, coronal section, shows the severe loss of tissue from a chronic MCA territory stroke (F). Pathology courtesy of Robert Schmidt MD, PhD.

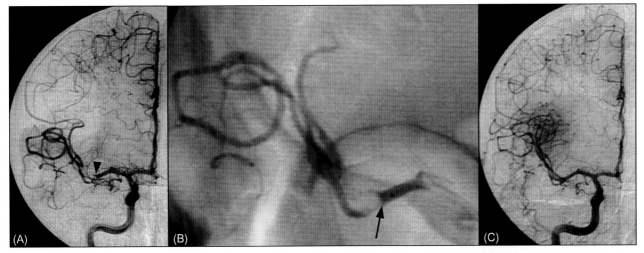

3.18 Distal MCA occlusion, recanalized. This lesion, a saddle embolus at the branch point of the distal superior M2 division, is shown on conventional angiography: pre-treatment (arrowhead) (A); microcatheter injection isolates this lesion (arrow) (B); and post-treatment (C), with resumption of M2 flow into the parietal lobe.

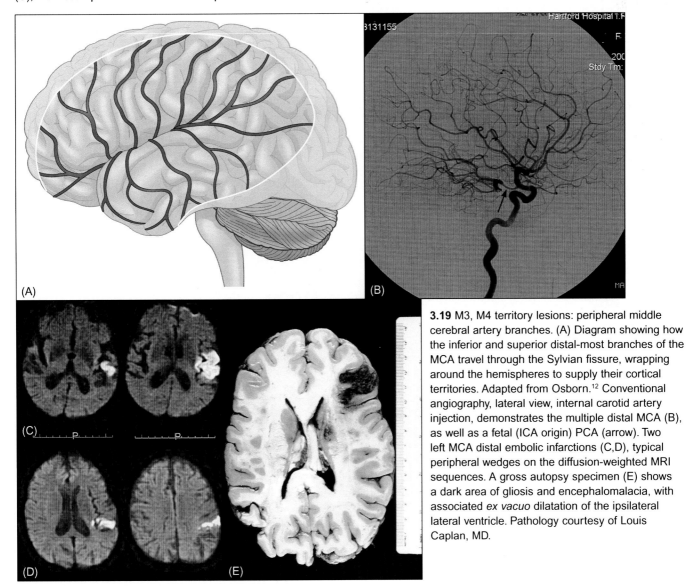

3.19 M3, M4 territory lesions: peripheral middle cerebral artery branches. (A) Diagram showing how the inferior and superior distal-most branches of the MCA travel through the Sylvian fissure, wrapping around the hemispheres to supply their cortical territories. Adapted from Osborn.[12] Conventional angiography, lateral view, internal carotid artery injection, demonstrates the multiple distal MCA (B), as well as a fetal (ICA origin) PCA (arrow). Two left MCA distal embolic infarctions (C,D), typical peripheral wedges on the diffusion-weighted MRI sequences. A gross autopsy specimen (E) shows a dark area of gliosis and encephalomalacia, with associated *ex vacuo* dilatation of the ipsilateral lateral ventricle. Pathology courtesy of Louis Caplan, MD.

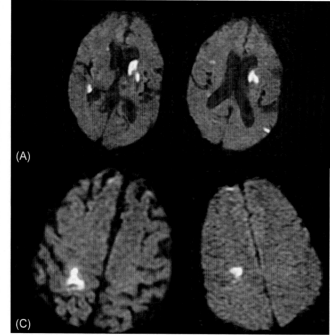

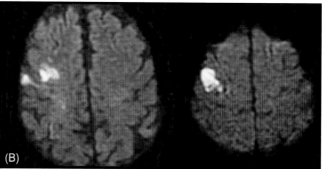

3.20 Distal, peripheral emboli. Bihemispheric emboli (A) indicate a cardiac or aortic rather than a unilateral carotid source. Individual small thromboemboli typically create lesions in gyral patterns (B; and C, left), or watershed territories (C, right) (see also **3.6**A,B).

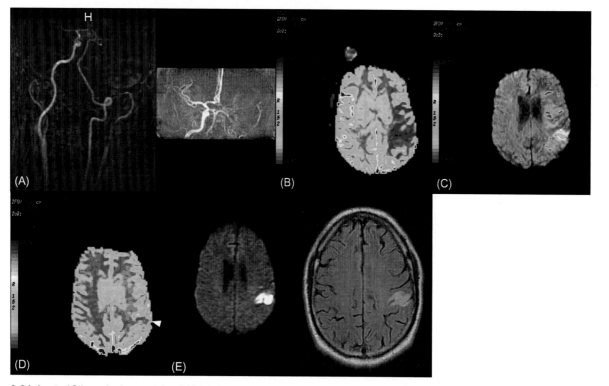

3.21 Acute ICA occlusion causing MCA infarction. MRA documents a left cervical ICA occlusion, coronal image (A, left), with poor intracranial MCA flow (A, right). Though a wide region of hypoperfusion is suggested by the perfusion CT scan (cerebral blood flow (B) and mean transit time (C) studies), a smaller eventual infarct size is suggested by a relatively smaller area of reduced cerebral blood volume (arrowhead) (D). Subsequent MRI scan demonstrated a small cortical-branch infarct in the parietal lobe (diffusion-weighted MRI (E, left) and FLAIR (E, right) sequences). The stroke etiology was likely 'stump embolism' from the ICA occlusion.

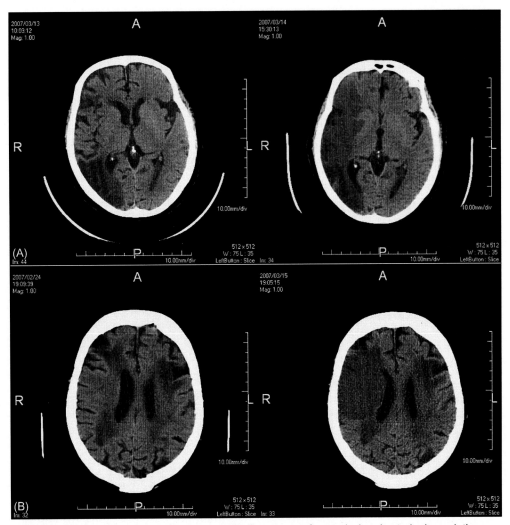

3.22 Old versus new stroke on CT scans (A,B). Two cases of acute ischemic stroke in evolution adjacent to earlier, old strokes. The new lesions (right images, in the anterior right hemispheres) are less hypodense, with associated early edema, while the older lesions demonstrate encephalomalacia (same density as cerebrospinal fluid).

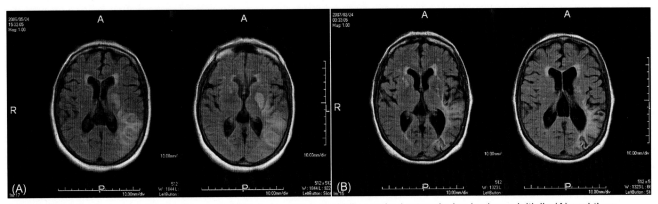

3.23 An acute lesion goes chronic. An acute M2 inferior-division middle cerebral artery lesion is shown initially (A) and then 9 months later (B) on serial FLAIR MRI sequences. Notice how the edema of early injured brain parenchyma develops into areas of cortical laminar necrosis.

*Symptoms of complete M1 occlusion (**3.14**)*
- Contralateral hemiplegia/paresis, sensory loss, and gaze palsy (causing gaze preference to the side of the stroke).
- Left M1 occlusion: global aphasia. *Note*: rarely, there is right hemisphere dominance for speech.
- Right M1 occlusion: left hemispatial neglect.
- Lesions involving >50% of MCA distribution have a high risk for development of the malignant MCA syndrome, with impending herniation during days 2–5 post-onset, heralded by a declining level of consciousness.

*Symptoms of superior division M2 occlusion (**3.17**, **3.18**)*
- Contralateral paresis and sensory loss of face and arm greater than that of the leg. The leg is represented more medially along the motor strip, in the parasagittal territory of the ACA.
- Contralateral gaze palsy.
- Left hemisphere: Broca's (expressive, non-fluent) aphasia.
- Right hemisphere: spatial neglect.

*Symptoms of inferior division M2 occlusion (**3.17**)*
- Contralateral superior quadrantic (or hemianopic) visual loss.
- Left hemisphere: Wernicke's (receptive, fluent) aphasia.
- Right hemisphere: spatial neglect.
- Note the lack of motor or sensory impairment in this distribution, making this a more difficult stroke to diagnose. Patients with Wernicke's aphasia may be misinterpreted as being confused, but the association with the visual field defect clarifies this as a stroke syndrome.

*Symptoms of more distal occlusions (**3.19**, **3.20**, **3.21**)*
The sensory or motor deficits are patchy, and most often affect the face and/or arm/hand because these body parts have large representation in the homunculus. Conversely, more proximal, subcortical, or brainstem lesions usually cause a more uniform hemiparesis of face, arm, and leg due to the tight collection of descending motor tracts. Diffusion-weighted MRI is the best modality to detect these smaller lesions in the acute phase.

Anterior cerebral artery territory

ACA strokes are much less common than MCA strokes because of the preferred pathway of emboli from the ICA into its larger and more direct extension, the MCA, and because an intact anterior communicating artery provides a source of collateral circulation to the ACA. The chief determinants of lesion size are how proximal within the ACA distribution the occlusion occurs and how wide this artery's territory extends, based upon the anatomy of the adjacent MCA and the ACA–MCA leptomeningeal collateral circulation. Several conventional angiographic studies show the ACA in anteroposterior (**3.11A**, **3.17**C, **3.18**A,C) and lateral (**3.8**C, **3.19**B) views.

Perforating branches

The most proximal perforator branches of the A1 and A2 (**3.13**, **3.24**) segments supply the head of the caudate nucleus, part of the basal ganglia and internal capsule, the anterior commissure, and the rostrum of the corpus callosum. The largest and longest ACA penetrating branch, the recurrent artery of Heubner, usually originates from the A2 segment and mostly supplies the head of the caudate (**3.13**, **3.24**; Chapter 2, **2.4**A). The medial lenticulostriate arteries and callosal perforating branches originating from A1 and A2 supply the anterobasal forebrain, corpus callosum genu, septum pellucidum, and fornix (**3.24**, **3.25**; Chapter 2, **2.5**A,D).

Cortical branches

The orbitofrontal branches supply the olfactory bulb and tract, the gyrus rectus, and the medial orbital gyrus while the frontopolar arteries supply the ventromedial frontal lobe and the corpus callosum (**3.26**–**3.29**).

Symptoms of anterior cerebral artery stroke[16,17]
- Contralateral weakness and sensory loss involving the leg to a much greater degree than the arm and face. This is the opposite pattern of the motor impairment seen in MCA strokes. Small emboli to the ACA territory may present with only intermittent 'TIAs' with contralateral leg paresis (**3.28**).
- Transient expressive aphasia may occur.
- If bilateral ACA strokes occur, frontal lobe symptoms such as flattened affect and depression, lack of interest and initiative, and cognitive impairment occur in addition to bilateral leg weakness (paraparesis) or paralysis (paraplegia) (**3.29**).

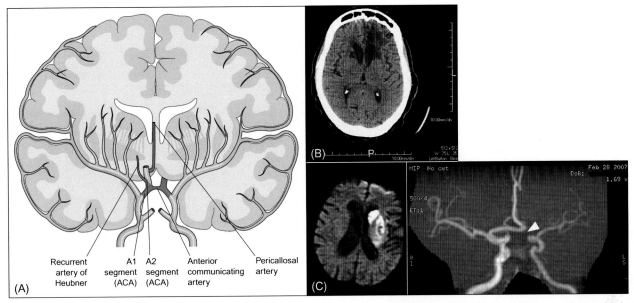

3.24 ACA anatomy and infarcts in the distribution of the recurrent artery of Heubner. A coronal illustration demonstrates the large vessels around the proximal ACA and circle of Willis. Adapted with permission from Osborn.[16] Note lesions to the head of the caudate nuclei bilaterally, with extensive damage to the left frontal lobe, on a CT scan (B). A second case (C, left) involves not only the territory of the recurrent artery of Heubner, but also lenticulostriate branches of the MCA. On MRA (C, right), the left A1 segment, where the artery of Heubner most commonly originates, appears absent or occluded (arrowhead).

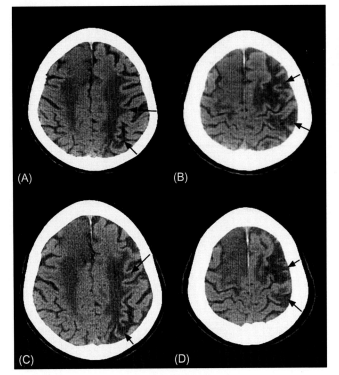

3.26 Acute right ACA infarct on serial CTs. The earlier scans (A,B) were obtained about 24 hours prior to the later ones (C,D) and demonstrate early right frontal lobe edema. Note subtle blunting of the right parasagittal and frontal sulci (A,B) compared with the contralateral hemisphere. An old hypodensity is also present in the left hemisphere in the ACA–MCA borderzone (arrows).

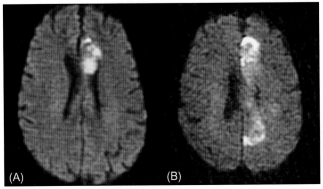

3.25 ACA infarction of proximal and perforator territories. These diffusion-weighted MRI studies in two patients show proximal ACA infarcts, with involvement of the corpus callosum (both anterior and posterior components in (B)) and mass effect upon the lateral ventricle.

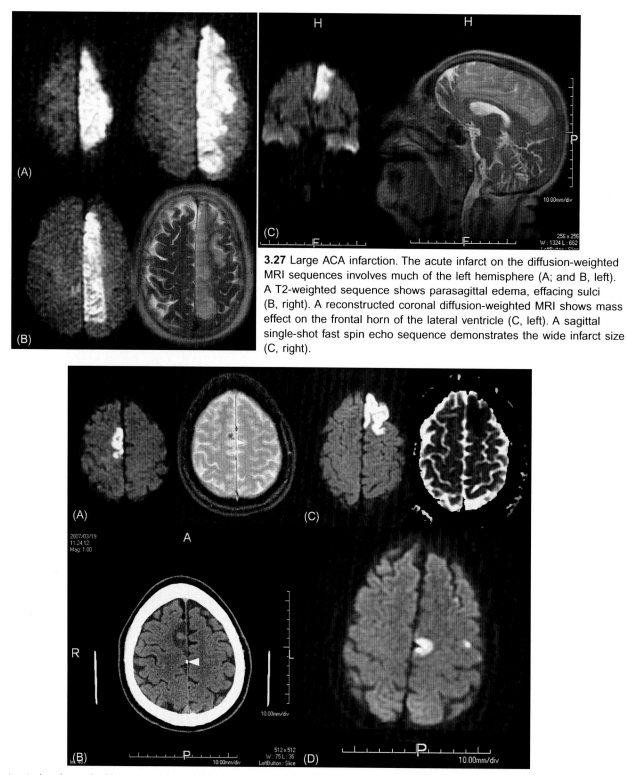

3.27 Large ACA infarction. The acute infarct on the diffusion-weighted MRI sequences involves much of the left hemisphere (A; and B, left). A T2-weighted sequence shows parasagittal edema, effacing sulci (B, right). A reconstructed coronal diffusion-weighted MRI shows mass effect on the frontal horn of the lateral ventricle (C, left). A sagittal single-shot fast spin echo sequence demonstrates the wide infarct size (C, right).

3.28 Acute strokes in cortical branches of the ACA. A small right ACA-distribution embolic stroke (diffusion-weighted MRI sequence (A, left, and GE MRI sequence, right)), with mild hemorrhagic transformation and calcified falx cerebri (arrowhead) on head CT scan (B). Restricted diffusion (diffusion-weighted MRI) of a second lesion is shown (C, left), with its accompanying apparent diffusion coefficient map (C, right). A third case shows punctuate embolic strokes in the left ACA and more lateral MCA territories on diffusion-weighted MRI (D).

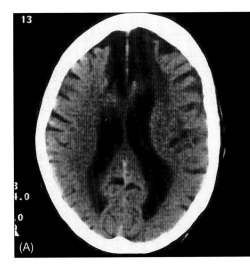
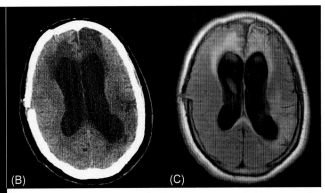

3.29 Bilateral ACA infarctions. Two CT scans of chronic, bilateral frontal lobe infarcts, the first from multifocal cardiogenic emboli (A) and a second due to complications of the surgical clipping of an intracranial aneurysm of the ACoA (B, and C, a FLAIR MRI sequence). An old left parietal (MCA territory) infarct is also present (B,C).

Case studies

Case study 1. Common carotid and M1 occlusions: intravenous thrombolysis and endovascular approaches

History

A 59-year-old woman was at home when she presented with new-onset speech difficulty and right hemiparesis. Her daughter witnessed the event, and called '911' within minutes. Her NIHSS score on arrival in the emergency department, 50 minutes after symptoms onset, was 22 points.

Timeline

Hospital day (HD) 1

1 *Emergent management:*

   05:30am   Onset of symptoms

05:47   Daughter calls EMS.

06:06   Stroke Team pager activated.

06:19   Arrival at Triage Desk:
- Emergency Department Evaluation.

06:40   Completed CT, CT angiography and CT perfusion studies (**CS 1.1**).

- A hyperdense left MCA sign (indicating the presence of a clot) is present on the initial CT scan (arrow) (A).
- The region of hypoperfusion is evident on the CT perfusion cerebral blood flow map (B), and prolonged mean transit time (C) as blue regions; however, cerebral blood volume (D) by contrast appears relatively normal, suggesting a cerebral blood flow–cerebral blood volume mismatch and indicating viable penumbra.

07:00   Intravenous tissue plasminogen activator (t-PA) bolus started (0.9 mg/kg, 10% bolus) = 8 mg bolus and 73 mg infusion:

- Door-to-drug time = 41 minutes.

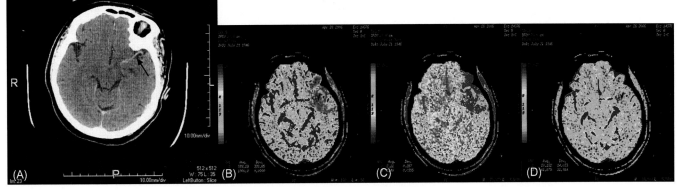

CS 1.1

07:30   The patient's daughter was consented for participation in the Multi-MERCI clinical trial.

2 *Endovascular procedures*:

07–8:00   Mobilization of the Interventional Neuro-radiology (INR) Team.

08:00   Patient transfer from emergency department to INR Suite.

08:15   Elective intubation, for endovascular procedure. (*Note*: some INR teams routinely use general anesthesia for endovascular procedures, while others do not so that the patient's neurological exam can be clinically monitored during the procedure).

08:30   Diagnostic conventional cerebral angiography (**CS 1.2**):

- Wide left common carotid artery/ICA occlusion (not shown).
- The primary lesion responsible for this stroke syndrome is a distal left M1 occlusion (arrows), shown on right ICA injection, late phase (A). Note the cross-filling via the anterior communicating artery, the hyperemia within the lenticulostriate system (arrowheads), and some early leptomeningeal collaterals to the left parietal region from the left ACA circulation (circled region).
- Other collateralization is appreciated on a left vertebral artery injection, late phase (B), with some left PCA flow supplying left MCA territory (circle).

09:37   The first two attempted Multi-MERCI LX device passes failed to remove any thrombus from within the M1 occlusion. The image shows a non-subtracted view with the MERCI device in the M1 segment, immediately behind the upper margin of the orbit on an antero-posterior projection (**CS 1.2C**).

10:33   Intra-arterial t-PA infusion (**CS 1.3**):

- Traversing the anterior communicating artery, via a right carotid approach (A, unsubtracted; B, subtracted image), with thrombolytic infusion into the local thrombus (arrows) (B). Note how the microcatheter must make a sharp 180-degree turn at the distal right ICA into the adjacent A1 segment (arrowhead) in order to access the anterior communicating artery and then advance into the contralateral, left M1 occlusion.

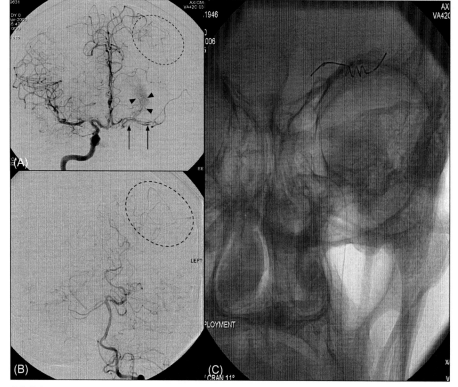

CS 1.2

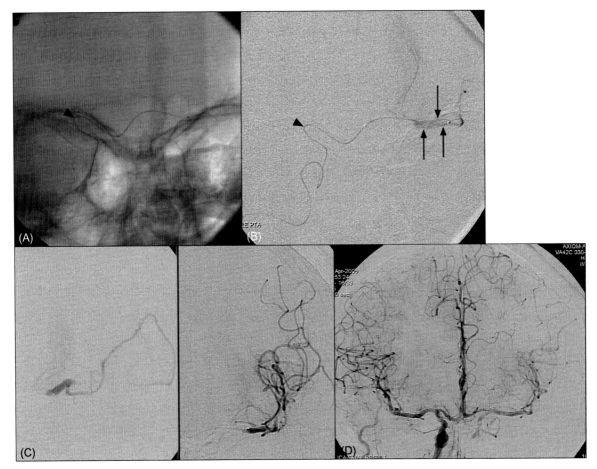

CS 1.3

- 10-mg intra-arterial t-PA bolus was injected directly into the M1 occlusion; subsequent 14-mg intra-arterial infusion over 1 hour 10 minutes. Microcatheter infusion demonstrates ongoing, partial recanalization of M1 lesion over time (B,C). A post-infusion injection into the right ICA shows improved flow to much of the left hemisphere (MCA territory) (D). Compare this post-infusion image (**CS 1.3D**) to the pre-treatment study (**CS 1.2A**).

  12:00   The procedure concluded, and patient is transferred to the ICU.

3 *Hospital course and clinical follow-up.*
HD 2
- Extubated.
- NIHSS = 3 points: expressive aphasia, with right facial and arm paresis.
- Brain MRI, diffusion-weighted image sequence (**CS 1.4**),

documents small, predominantly subcortical, patchy lesions within the left MCA territory (A,B).

HD 3
- Transferred out of the ICU.
- Warfarin started to prevent recurrent emboli from the common carotid artery/ICA occlusion.

HD 4
- The patient begins to complain of 'blurry vision' in her left eye (OS).
- Her neurologic exam, other than partial loss of vision OS, has normalized.
- NIHSS = 1 point: monocular visual loss.

HD 5
- Transfer to acute rehabilitation.
- She returns to home 5 days later.

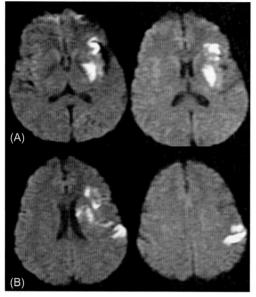

CS 1.4

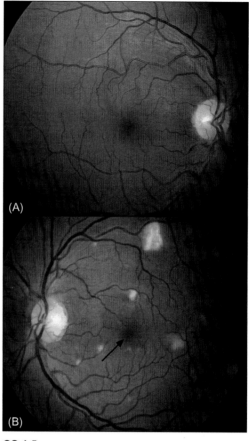

CS 1.5

30-day outpatient follow-up

- Funduscopic photos (**CS 1.5**) document a normal right eye (A) but multiple branch retinal emboli in the left eye (B), explaining her visual deficit.
- Much of her visual loss improved, because the fovea (arrow) was largely spared from ischemic injury (B).

Comments

This patient's NIHSS score of >20 points would carry a high risk for developing a large MCA stroke, with greater than 90% likelihood of post-stroke death or severe disability.[18] Factors influencing a favorable outcome included: (1) the early time to arrival at the emergency department and rapid processing, facilitating early exposure to IV t-PA; (2) interventional expertise to access the lesion, via the contralateral ICA, by traversing an intact anterior communicating artery; and (3) the patient's recruitment of leptomeningeal hemispheric collaterals, suggested by the initial CT perfusion study and subsequent conventional angiography.

This patient's management was aggressive, in that multiple attempts at endovascular recanalization were made following intravenous thrombolysis. Her sole morbidity, partial visual loss OS, was due to thromboembolism into the central retinal artery from the ICA thrombus via its first intracranial branch, the ophthalmic artery. The hemispheric stroke, by contrast, caused no functional limitations.

The emergent treatment of tandem lesions (here, common carotid artery/ICA and MCA occlusions) is evolving. An alternative endovascular approach would have been angioplasty with or without stent placement across the common carotid/ICA occlusion, and then advancing the catheter directly upstream to the MCA occlusion.

References

1. Tatu L, Moulin T, Bogousslavsky J, Duvernoy H. Arterial territories of human brain: brainstem and cerebellum. *Neurology* 1996; **47**: 1125–35.
2. Tatu L, Moulin T, Bogousslavsky J, Duvernoy H. Arterial territories of the human brain: cerebral hemispheres. *Neurology* 1998; **50**: 1699–708.
3. Osborn A. The Circle of Willis. In: *Diagnostic Cerebral Angiography*, 2nd edn. Philadelphia, PA: Lippincott Williams & Wilkins; 1999: 105–16.
4. Liebeskind D. Collateral circulation. *Stroke* 2003; **34**: 2279–84.

5. Osborn A. Atherosclerosis and carotid stenosis. In: *Diagnostic Cerebral Angiography*, 2nd edn. Philadelphia, PA: Lippincott Williams & Wilkins; 1999: 359–79.

6. Saver J, Biller J. Superficial middle cerebral artery. In: Bogousslavsky J, Caplan L, eds. *Stroke Syndromes*. New York: Cambridge University; 1995: 247–59.

7. Bogousslavsky J, Moulin T. Border-zone infarcts. In: Bogousslavsky J, Caplan L, eds. *Stroke Syndromes*. New York: Cambridge University; 1995: 358–66.

8. Osborn A. The internal carotid artery: cavernous, clinoid, ophthalmic and communicating segments. In: *Diagnostic Cerebral Angiography*, 2nd edn. Philadelphia, PA: Lippincott Williams & Wilkins; 1999: 83–104.

9. Osborn A. The internal carotid artery: cervical, petrous, and lacerum segments. In: *Diagnostic Cerebral Angiography*, 2nd edn. Philadelphia, PA: Lippincott Williams & Wilkins; 1999: 57–81.

10. Wray S. Visual symptoms (eye). In: Bogousslavsky J, Caplan L, eds. *Stroke Syndromes*, 2nd edn. New York: Cambridge University Press; 2001: 111–28.

11. Helgason C. Anterior choroidal artery. In: Bogousslavsky J, Caplan L, eds. *Stroke Syndromes*. New York: Cambridge University; 1995: 270–6.

12. Osborn A. The middle cerebral artery. In: *Diagnostic Cerebral Angiography*, 2nd edn. Philadelphia, PA: Lippincott Williams & Wilkins; 1999: 135–52.

13. Vahedi K, Hofmeijer J, Juettler E, *et al.* Early decompressive surgery in malignant infarction of the middle cerebral artery: a pooled analysis of three randomised controlled trials. *Lancet* 2007; **6**: 215–22.

14. Phan T, Donnan G, Wright P, Reutens D. A digital map of middle cerebral artery infarcts associated with middle cerebral artery trunk and branch occlusion. *Stroke* 2005; **36**: 986–91.

15. Kumral E, Ozdemirkiran T, Alper Y. Strokes in the subinsular territory: clinical, topographical, and etiological patterns. *Neurology* 2004; **63**: 2429–32.

16. Osborn A. The anterior cerebral artery. In: *Diagnostic Cerebral Angiography*, 2nd edn. Philadelphia, PA: Lippincott Williams & Wilkins; 1999: 117–35.

17. Sawada T, Kazui S. Anterior cerebral artery. In: Bogousslavsky J, Caplan L, eds. *Stroke Syndromes*. New York: Cambridge University; 1995: 235–46.

18. Adams HP Jr, Davis P, Leira E, *et al.* Baseline NIH Stroke Scale score strongly predicts outcome after stroke: a report of the Trial of Org 10172 in Acute Stroke Treatment (TOAST). *Neurology* 1999; **53**: 126–31.

Further reading

Bogousslavsky J, Caplan L. *Stroke Syndromes*, 2nd edn. New York: Cambridge University Press; 2001.

Liebeskind D. Collateral circulation. *Stroke* 2003; **34**: 2279–84.

Osborn A. *Diagnostic Neuroradiology*, 2nd edn. St Louis, MO: Mosby; 1994.

Tatu L, Moulin T, Bogousslavsky J, Duvernoy H. Arterial territories of the human brain: cerebral hemispheres. *Neurology* 1998; **50**: 1699–708.

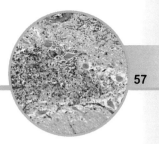

Chapter 4

Posterior Circulation

Introduction: anatomy

The posterior circulation, the vertebrobasilar system, receives 20% of the blood flow to the brain and supplies the brainstem, cerebellum, and most of the temporal and occipital lobes (**4.1**). Two vertebral arteries (VA) converge to form the basilar artery (BA). This is the only place in the body where two arteries converge rather than branch,

enabling some redundancy.[1,2] If one VA is occluded proximal to the posterior inferior cerebellar artery (PICA), the other vertebral may provide retrograde collateral flow to the PICA. Another unusual feature is that, in the neck, the VAs course through the C6 to C1 vertebral transverse foraminae. The bone provides some protection for the arteries; however, degenerative spine disease and traumatic dissection are potential causes for arterial injury (**4.1F**; Chapter 1, **1.2**).

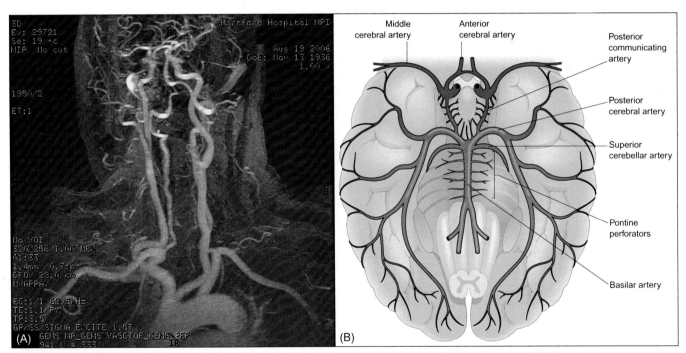

4.1 Vertebrobasilar anatomy. The cervical and intracranial vertebrobasilar system is shown on a coronal MRA sequence (A; Chapter 2, **2.1**A). The paired vertebral arteries have extraosseous, foraminal, extraspinal, and intradural segments that run from the cervical region, through the meninges, to their intracranial termination at the basilar junction.[1] The extracranial vertebral arteries may be difficult to fully appreciate on MRA due to the overlying carotid system (A). A view of the posterior circulation 'draped' over the ventral surface of the brainstem and cerebellar hemispheres (B): BA; posterior communicating artery (PCoA); PCA; superior cerebellar artery (SCA); pontine perforators.

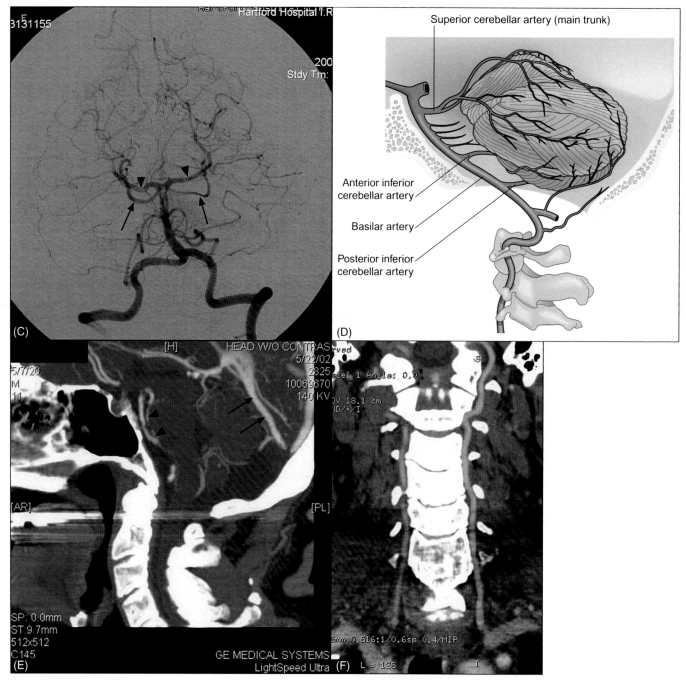

4.1 (*continued*) Vertebrobasilar anatomy. The distal vertebral arteries and the pontine perforator branches originating from the BA are shown on a conventional angiogram (anteroposterior, Townes' projection) (C); the SCA (arrows) and PCAs (arrowheads) are well visualized. A lateral view of the cerebellar hemisphere shows the three major cerebellar arteries (D). B and D adapted from Osborn.[1] CT scans with contrast: on a sagittal view (E), the relation of the arteries of the posterior circulation to the cerebellum and the proximity of the BA (arrowheads) to the clivus bone (anterior) are appreciated. Other contrast represents flow within the venous sinuses, such as the straight sinus (arrows). On a coronal view (F), the cervical vertebral arteries are seen to traverse the vertebral foramina.

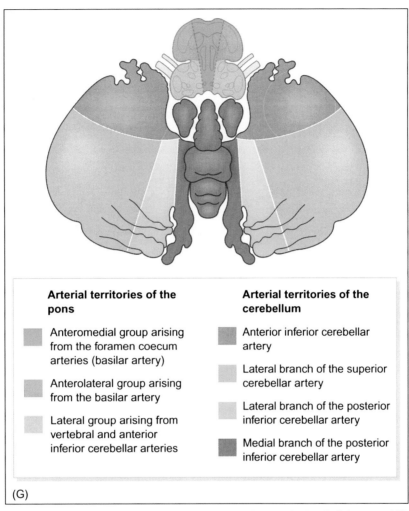

Arterial territories of the pons

▪ Anteromedial group arising from the foramen coecum arteries (basilar artery)

▪ Anterolateral group arising from the basilar artery

▪ Lateral group arising from vertebral and anterior inferior cerebellar arteries

Arterial territories of the cerebellum

▪ Anterior inferior cerebellar artery

▪ Lateral branch of the superior cerebellar artery

▪ Lateral branch of the posterior inferior cerebellar artery

▪ Medial branch of the posterior inferior cerebellar artery

(G)

4.1 (*continued*) Vertebrobasilar anatomy. An MRI-based map, transverse section, at the level of the pons (G), demonstrates the complexity of vascular territories within the posterior fossa. With permission from Tatu *et al.*[2]

Cerebellum and brainstem

The most common sites for the development of large vessel atherosclerotic disease in the posterior circulation are the branch points of the system at the proximal and distal ends of the VAs and at the distal end of the BA as it divides into the two PCAs (**case study 1**).[1]

Three paired cerebellar arteries (PICA anterior inferior, and superior) (**4.1D**) wrap around the cerebellar hemispheres.[3,4] Some smaller cerebellar infarcts are shown (**4.2**). The largest ischemic strokes in the cerebellar hemispheres are typically in the distribution of the PICA (**4.3**, **4.4**), and, like cerebellar hemorrhage, may require decompressive craniotomy to avoid death of the patient (**4.3**).

In addition to the cerebellar hemispheres (**4.2–4.4**), common sites for vertebrobasilar stroke include the paramedian pons (**4.5**) and the lateral medulla (**4.6**). The lateral pons (**4.7**) and the medial medulla (**4.8**) are uncommon locations. Distal embolic showers through the posterior circulation often produce multifocal lesions, particularly involving distal branches of the posterior circulation, into the PCA territories. The associated symptoms are often referred to as the 'top-of-the-basilar' syndrome (**4.9**).

Symptoms of vertebrobasilar stroke

The range of symptoms and signs is quite extensive and they can fluctuate widely over the initial few hours of presentation, making diagnosis potentially more complicated than in anterior circulation strokes. The complexity of neurologic

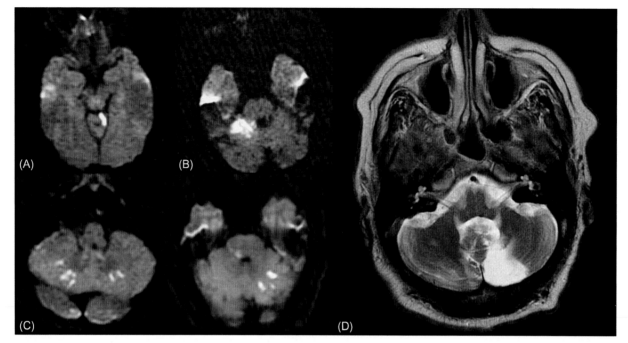

4.2 Cerebellar strokes. Small lesions in the medial and lateral cerebellar hemispheres on diffusion-weighted MRI sequences (A–C). A chronic infarct in the distribution of the medial branch of the left PICA is a wedge-shaped hyperintense area on MRI (T2WI) (D).

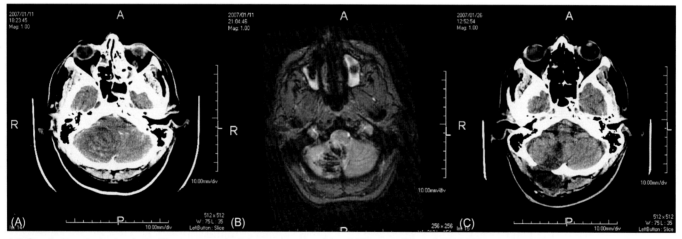

4.3 Cerebellar stroke treated with neurosurgical decompression. Head CT scan (A) and GE MRI sequence (B) show significant hemorrhagic transformation of a large right PICA distribution stroke, with effacement of the fourth ventricle and mass effect on the medulla. Postoperative CT scan obtained 7 days later demonstrates the recovery of the basal cisterns (C).

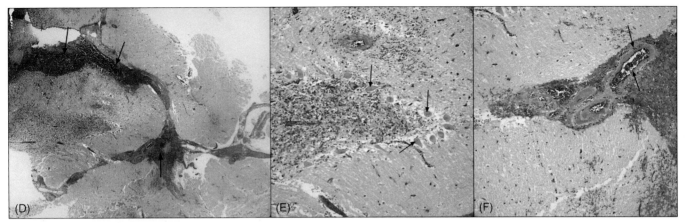

4.3 (*continued*) Cerebellar stroke treated with neurosurgical decompression. Micropathology of the resected lesion (hematoxylin and eosin stains) shows hemorrhage (red blood cells, arrows) above and within the pale, infarcted cerebellar tissue (D, 10×). Magnified views (40×) of the tissue show swollen, newly dead Purkinje fibers (arrows) (E) and arteriosclerotic (thickened) arterial walls (arrows) (F), consistent with long-standing hypertension. Pathology courtesy of Dean Uphoff, MD.

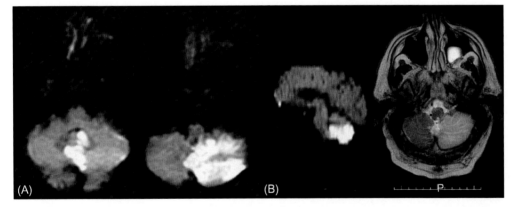

4.4 Infarction of the left PICA. Diffusion-weighted MRI (A) and FLAIR MRI (B, right) sequences, as well as a reconstructed sagittal diffusion-weighted MRI sequence (B, left) shows that PICA supplies the inferior half of the cerebellar hemisphere.

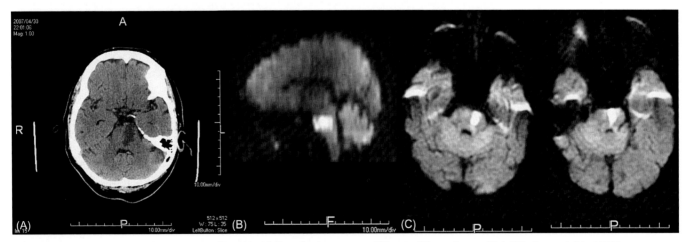

4.5 Paramedian pontine stroke. A large left pontine infarct is shown on a CT scan (A), and a sagittal diffusion-weighted MRI sequence (B). Diffusion-weighted MRI sequences of two smaller infarctions in the distribution of the left paramedian pontine perforators (C) affect primarily the medial motor tracts. (The heightened signal in the bilateral medial temporal lobes (C) is artifactual.)

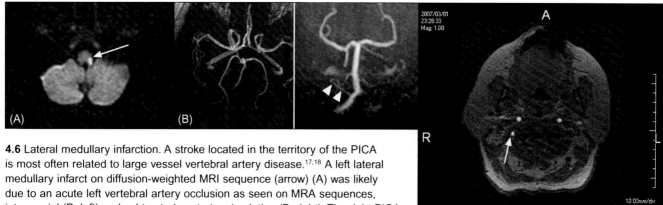

4.6 Lateral medullary infarction. A stroke located in the territory of the PICA is most often related to large vessel vertebral artery disease.[17,18] A left lateral medullary infarct on diffusion-weighted MRI sequence (arrow) (A) was likely due to an acute left vertebral artery occlusion as seen on MRA sequences, intracranial (B, left) and subtracted posterior circulation (B, right). The right PICA is well visualized (arrowheads), while the left PICA is not. Transaxial source images for this MRA show no signal (flow) in the left vertebral artery, in contrast to the right vertebral artery (arrow) (C).

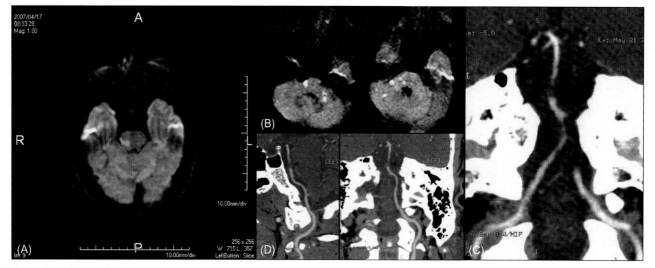

4.7 Lateral pontine and cerebellar strokes. An isolated right lateral pontine infarct is shown on diffusion-weighted MRI (A). A second patient presented with bilateral hearing loss, varying sensory symptoms, and gait imbalance. The responsible embolic lesions primarily affected bilateral anterior inferior cerebellar artery (AICA) territories in the pons, lateral cerebellum, and cerebellar peduncles on the diffusion-weighted MRI sequences (B). On a CT scan with contrast, atherostenotic lesions are present in the distal left VA and the proximal and mid-BA (C). However, on focused sagittal (D, left) and coronal (D, right) windowing, the predominant area of stenosis, and the likely source of this stroke syndrome, is the mid-basilar artery disease (arrowheads).

deficits is amplified when parts of the brainstem are involved in addition to the cerebellum.[5] They include:

- gait or limb ataxia (patients often fall towards or veer towards the side of the lesion, when ambulating; or have ipsilateral limb ataxia);
- midline or medial cerebellar lesions may only cause gait imbalance and vestibular symptoms, with no or minimal limb ataxia;[6]
- nystagmus;
- diplopia, horizontal or vertical;
- vertigo, tinnitus, hearing loss;
- nausea and vomiting;
- variable patterns of limb weakness and sensory loss;
- dysarthria and dysphagia.

In general, the positioning of nuclei and tracts within the brainstem dictate that motor (limb and oculomotor) deficits correspond to more medial lesions, while sensory and ataxic symptoms result from more lateral lesions.

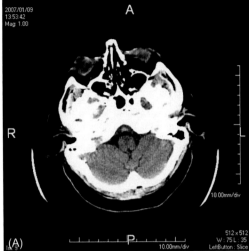
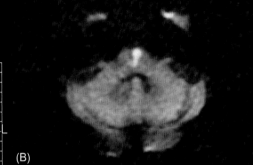

4.8 Medial medullary infarction. A CT scan barely registers the lesion (A), shown readily on a diffusion-weighted MRI sequence (B). The etiologies of medial medullary infarction include large and small vessel atherosclerotic disease and vertebral artery dissection.[17]

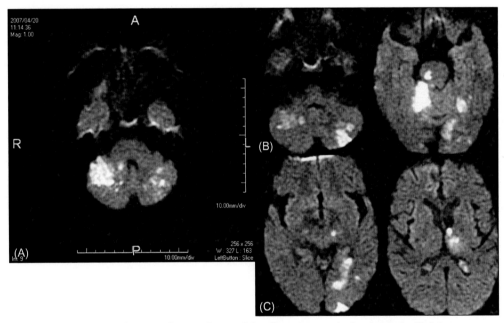

4.9 Distal emboli: top-of-the-basilar syndrome. A basilar artery occlusion treated with intravenous and then intra-arterial thrombolysis, with significant recanalization. The diffusion-weighted MRI sequences (A–C) document patchy, multifocal lesions throughout the posterior circulation, involving the cerebellar hemispheres, pons, midbrain, occipital lobes, and thalamus.[3]

Most important in evaluating the acute stroke patient is simply to localize the patient's symptoms to the posterior circulation rather than to a specific arterial distribution, as this determines the diagnostic work-up: screening for potential lesions of the VA or BA and embolic sources from the vertebrobasilar tree, the aorta, and the heart.[5] Owing to bony artifact in the posterior fossa on CT imaging, MRI is the preferred modality for identifying infarcts in the posterior circulation.

Basilar artery territory

Occlusion of the BA (**4.10**, **4.11**) are the location of the greatest concern in the posterior circulation. Untreated, BA occlusion carries a 50–80% mortality rate in case series.[7] The high morbidity and mortality reflects the basilar artery's supply to autonomic centers of the brainstem as well as the paramedian major motor tracts.[8,9] If the patient survives, a 'locked-in' syndrome is not uncommon. In this situation, the patient may be alert and awake but cannot move with the exception of eye blinking and eye movement. Anatomically, the dorsal brainstem (afferent tracts) is intact and the ventral brainstem (efferent tracts) has infarcted.

By contrast, recanalization of a BA occlusion with mechanical embolectomy or thrombolysis is associated with favorable outcomes in a significant percentage of patients (**case study 2**). The top-of-the-basilar syndrome occurs when there is occlusion of the distal or rostral portion of the BA usually by an embolus. Clinical presentation includes change in level of consciousness, visual symptoms, including hallucinations or blindness, oculomotor and pupillary abnormalities, with or without motor symptoms such as decerebrate posturing.

Posterior cerebral artery territory

The PCAs are the distal-most branches of the vertebrobasilar system (**4.1**). The two most common stroke etiologies are emboli into one or both PCA branches, originating from large vessel atherosclerosis in one of the VAs or within the heart, and small vessel disease affecting the deep perforating branches of the PCAs.[3,10,11] In contrast with the middle cerebral artery, proximal PCA atherostenosis is uncommon.

Perforating branches (**4.12**A)

The first two segments of the PCA, the P1 (pre-communicating) and P2 (ambient) segments, provide local perforator branches to the thalamus, hypothalamus, the posterior limb of the internal capsule, the midbrain, and rostral cranial–nerve nuclei (oculomotor and trochlear nerves).[10]

The etiology of infarcts involving the central penetrating branches (the thalamoperforating, thalamogeniculate, and peduncular perforating arteries) is small vessel disease

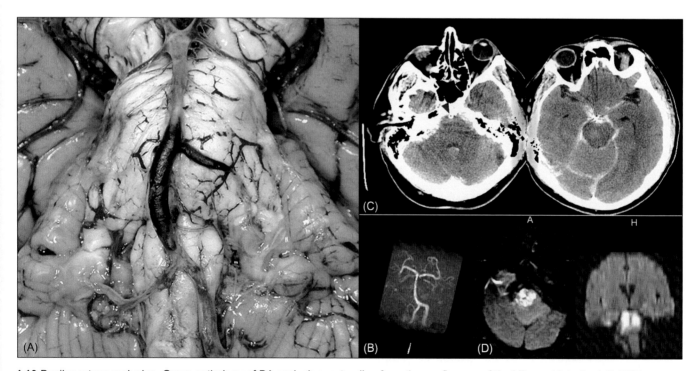

4.10 Basilar artery occlusion. Gross pathology of BA occlusion, extending from the confluence of the VAs and into the left AICA. Pathology courtesy of Louis Caplan, MD. A case of BA occlusion treated with a multimodal approach. A stent, placed in the BA, appears as a fence-like structure in the post-procedural intracranial MRA (B). On CT scan (C), the stent is seen as a hyperdense circle (arrowhead) (left) and metallic artifact with significant subarachnoid hemorrhage (right). Despite excellent recanalization, transaxial (D, left) and reconstructed coronal diffusion-weighted MRI (D, right) sequences document bilateral pontine infarction.

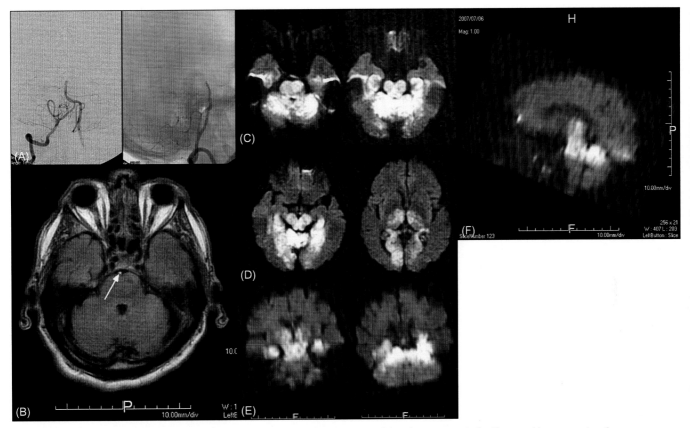

4.11 Basilar artery occlusion, following failed recanalization. This 70-year-old patient presented with a rapid progression from hemiparesis to quadriparesis, diminished level of consciousness, small and poorly reactive pupils, acute respiratory failure, and bilateral Babinski signs. Urgent angiography documented distal BA occlusion, but endovascular attempts were unsuccessful. Conventional angiography, right vertebral artery injection (A), shows the final appearance of the occluded mid-BA on anteroposterior (left) and lateral (right) projections. The MRI study on the following day shows hyperintense signal on the FLAIR sequence within the BA (arrow) (B). The massive infarct on DW-MRI sequence, transaxial (C,D), coronal (E), and sagittal (F) images, encompasses the territories of the BA perforators, plus the bilateral SCA and PCA territories: the pons and midbrain, the rostral cerebellum and vermis, occipital lobes, and thalamus.

(Chapter 2, **2.6**). Multifocal lesions in this region can also be embolic; e.g., part of a top-of-the-basilar syndrome (**4.9**).[12]

Cortical branches (4.12B)

The more proximal occipital artery (lateral branch of the PCA) supplies most of the temporal lobe, particularly the inferomedial temporal region. The more distal medial occipital artery (posterior, medial branch of the PCA) supplies the occipital lobe, including the primary calcarine (visual) cortex and often the adjacent parieto-occipital region. A variety of cortical PCA lesions is shown (**4.12–4.16**).

The fetal posterior cerebral artery variant (4.17)

Frequently, the PCA does not develop into a distal branch of the BA, but remains a fetal remnant in which it continues as an extension of the ICA. The so-called 'fetal PCA' is the most common variant of the cervical and intracranial arterial territories, and occurs unilaterally in 5–10% of all individuals.[10] With this anatomy, the proximal PCA is larger than the adjacent posterior communicating artery, and symptomatic carotid atherosclerotic disease may embolize into an ipsilateral fetal PCA as well as middle cerebral artery and anterior cerebral artery territories (Chapter 3).[13]

Symptoms of posterior cerebral artery stroke

The most prominent symptom of a cortical PCA stroke is usually a contralateral visual field deficit, a homonymous hemianopia or quadrantanopia. Central vision loss occurs when the occipital pole is involved. If bilateral PCA strokes

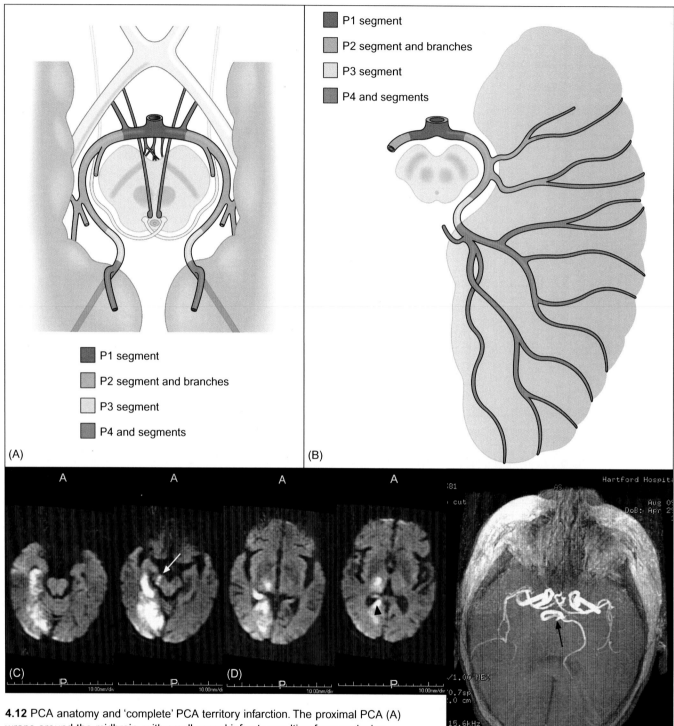

4.12 PCA anatomy and 'complete' PCA territory infarction. The proximal PCA (A) wraps around the midbrain, with small vessel infarcts resulting from occlusion of the perforators off the P1 and P2 segments and the PCoAs. A map of the cortical branches of the PCA (B), as they originate from the P2 and P3 segments. Adapted with permission from Osborn.[10] An acute infarct of the right P1 segment, demonstrating involvement of occipital lobe and medial temporal lobes (C,D), the cerebral peduncle (arrow) (C, right), and the thalamus (D) as well as the splenium of the corpus callosum (D, right; arrowhead). The lesion on transaxial MRA shows no flow into the right PCA (arrow) (E).

involving the occipital lobes occur, there may be cortical blindness.[3] However, PCA strokes are noteworthy for a wide range of other associated neurologic deficits, including memory impairment, visual agnosias, visuospatial processing difficulties, and visual hallucinations. When there is thalamic involvement, hemisensory loss, behavioral disorders and higher cognitive processing difficulties can occur and contribute to vascular dementia (**4.16**).[11,14–16]

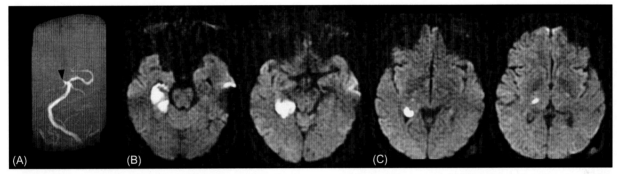

4.13 Smaller P1 segment infarct. A right P1 occlusion is shown on an isolated intracranial MRA of the posterior circulation (arrowhead) (A), while the more inferior SCA is intact. The infarct on diffusion-weighted magnetic MRI sequences involves the anteromedial temporal lobe (B), the choroidal region of the lateral ventricle (C, left), and thalamus (C, right).

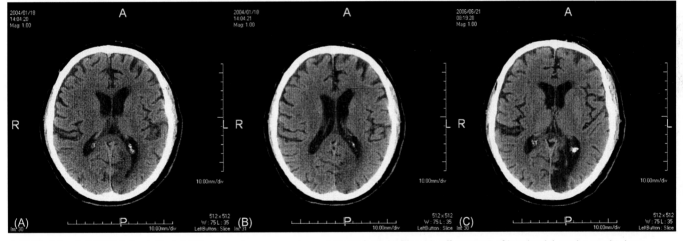

4.14 Evolving left PCA infarct. Serial CT scans show an acute occipital infarct (A,B), with effacement of local sulci, and a study done 2 years later (C). The associated encephalomalacia of the chronic lesion results in *ex vacuo* expansion of the adjacent lateral ventricle (C).

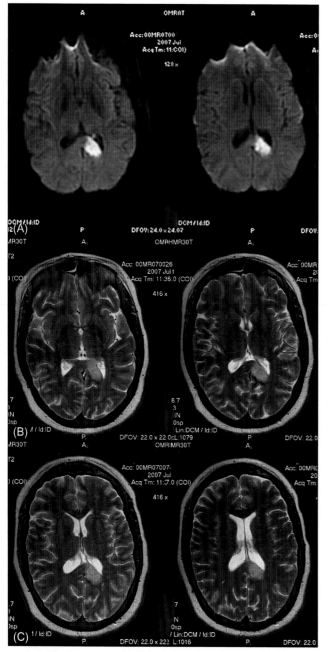

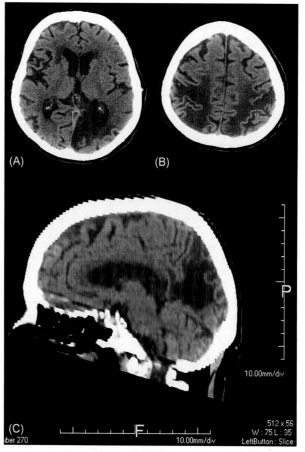

4.16 Vascular dementia with PCA infarction. Multiple old infarcts, including a left cortical PCA lesion (A). The thalamus is spared (A), but extensive encephalomalacia is seen in the frontoparietal regions, bilaterally (B). A reconstructed sagittal CT image illustrates how this lesion involves visual cortex in the medial occipital lobe (C).

4.15 Isolated infarct of the splenium. A 50-year-old woman presented with the acute onset of higher cognitive difficulties and memory impairment. The brain MRI scan documents an acute infarction of the left posterior corpus callosum on DW- (A) and T2-weighted (B-C) images.

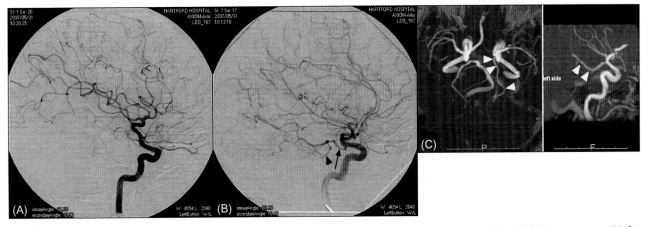

4.17 Fetal PCA anatomy. Lateral views of conventional angiography are compared in the same patient. (A) shows a normal left ICA injection, while the (B) shows a fetal PCA (arrow) originating from the right ICA. Another less common variant is a SCA (arrowhead) originating from the fetal PCA (B). In another patient, a MRA study demonstrates a left fetal PCA (C): a transaxial image demonstrates the left PCA (arrowheads) originating from the ICA (left). Note the lack of a P1 segment on that side. A sagittal MRA (right) isolating the anterior circulation also shows this fetal PCA (arrowheads).

Case studies

Case study 1. Vertebral artery stenting

This 65-year-old patient had recurrent posterior circulation ischemic events despite an aggressive cardiovascular medical regimen. The distal right VA has an irregular plaque, with a focal >50% stenosis, just proximal to a large PICA on a three-dimensional rendering of the conventional angiography

(**CS 1.1A**). The lesion was measured (**CS 1.1B**), and treated with balloon angioplasty and a Wingspan™ stent. On lateral projections (**CS 1.1C**), right VA injection images are shown before (left) and after stent placement (right), with some increase in the diameter of the lumen. An unsubtracted lateral view shows the relation of the treated VA to the skull base (**CS 1.1D**); the markers at ends of the stent consist of four radio-opaque points (an arrow is drawn to the proximal end).

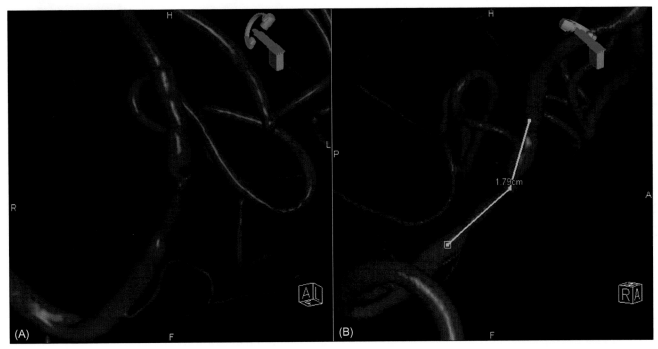

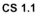

CS 1.1

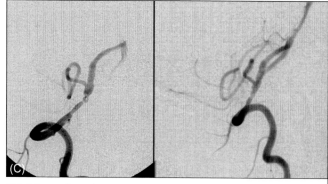

CS 1.1 *continued*

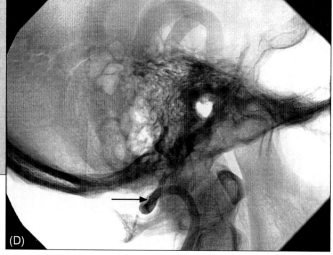

Comments

Typically, there is some asymmetry of the VAs. In this case, the dominant, or larger, right VA had severe atherosclerotic disease. The decision to treat with stenting was made because of recurrent TIAs as well as the severity of disease in this dominant VA.

Case study 2. Basilar artery occlusion, with late intra-arterial recanalization
History

A previously healthy 36-year-old woman presented with mild headache radiating to the occipital and cervical region for 2 days. Her only past medical history was of migraine headache and use of oral contraceptive agents. Her admission examination showed mild dysarthria, left facial paresis, and mild left arm ataxia. An urgent CT scan and lumbar puncture were normal, with the exception of a hyperdense BA (arrowhead) (**CS 2.1**), consistent with local thrombo-occlusive disease. The next morning, she developed worsening dysarthria and dysphagia, gaze paresis, difficulty managing secretions, and inability to generate cough, as well as increased ataxia in the left arm. An initial MRI scan (not shown) showed no major areas of diffusion abnormality. However, with the concern of a progressive posterior-circulation syndrome, the patient and her husband were consented for an endovascular intervention.

Intervention

Hospital day (HD) 2

- Diagnostic angiography (**CS 2.2**) showed a BA occlusion, with an abrupt cut-off in the proximal portion of the BA (arrows), possibly consistent with local dissection of this artery.
  - Views shown are unsubtracted (A), as well as subtracted earlier phase (B, left) and later phase (B, right)

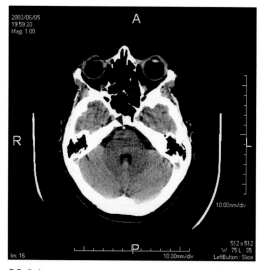

CS 2.1

anteroposterior left VA injection, demonstrating reflux back down the right distal VA.
- Anterior circulation injections of the right and left ICAs (shown side by side; C) also indicate that the BA occlusion encompasses much of this artery, as retrograde flow penetrates into only the distal-most portion of the BA (arrow).
- Intra-arterial (IA) thrombolysis (**CS 2.3**): IA tissue plasminogen activator (t-PA) 10 mg bolus with an additional 10 mg infusion over 1 hour.
  - Angiographic studies, lateral views (A–C), show progressive reopening of the local BA thrombus from the mid to distal BA.

Hospital course and clinical follow-up

- **HD3.** The post-procedural MRI scan (**CS 2.4**) the next day showed acute infarcts in the pons and adjacent cerebellar hemispheres, but a low overall lesion volume.
  - Diffusion-weighted (A; B, left) and FLAIR (B, right) MRI sequences are shown.
- **HD5.** The patient passed her swallow study.

- **HD7.** Mild left facial paresis and left arm ataxia.
  - Transfer to inpatient acute rehabilitation unit.
- **HD10.** Returns home.
- **3 weeks.** Returns to work.
- **30 days.** Outpatient follow-up, Neurovascular Clinic: asymptomatic.
- **90 days.** The patient e-mailed her vascular neurologist: 'Feeling altogether <u>normal</u>! Thank you.'

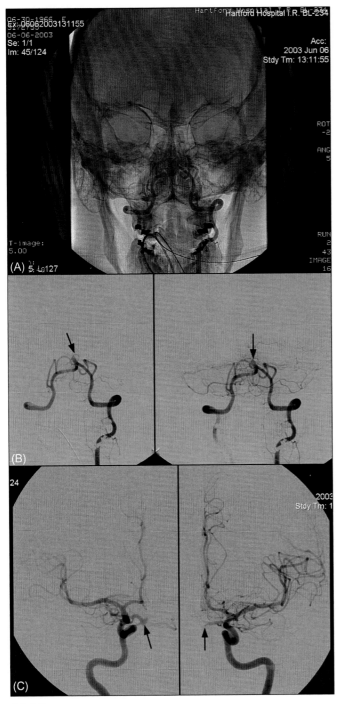

CS 2.2

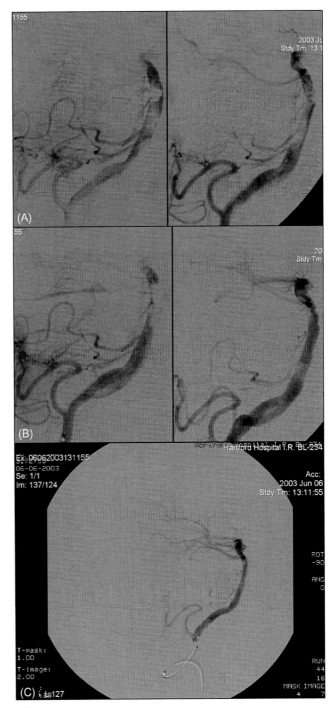

CS 2.3

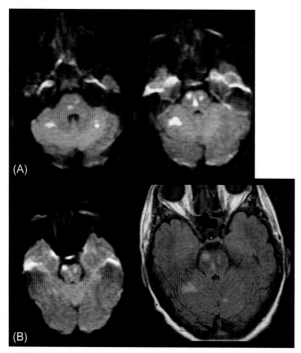

(A)

(B)

CS 2.4

Comments

This patient received IA thrombolysis starting 30 hours into her stroke syndrome, well beyond the traditional 3-hour window for intravenous t-PA and the 6-hour window for IA t-PA; she made a complete neurologic recovery. The brainstem is quite refractory to ischemia due to the tightly packed arterial system in this region and because it may access nearby extracranial (cervical) arteries for collateral circulation. Hence, case studies of IA thrombolysis for BA occlusion have been anecdotally successful 12–48 hours after symptom onset, particularly when, as in this case, a pre-procedural diffusion-weighted MRI sequence shows minimal-to-no infarction or a diffusion–perfusion mismatch.[19,20] In a systematic analysis comparing IA and intravenous thrombolysis for BA occlusion, recanalization rates were higher for the endovascular approach, at 65%, versus 53% for intravenous t-PA alone.[7]

References

1. Osborn A. The vertebrobasilar system. In: *Diagnostic Cerebral Angiography*, 2nd edn. Philadelphia, PA: Lippincott Williams & Wilkins; 1999: 173–94.

2. Tatu L, Moulin T, Bogousslavsky J, Duvernoy H. Arterial territories of human brain: brainstem and cerebellum. *Neurology* 1996; **47**: 1125–35.

3. Caplan L. Posterior cerebral artery. In: Bogousslavsky J, Caplan L, eds. *Stroke Syndromes*. New York: Cambridge University; 1995: 290–9.

4. Amarenco P. Cerebellar stroke syndromes. In: Bogousslavsky J, Caplan L, eds. *Stroke Syndromes*. New York: Cambridge University; 1995: 344–58.

5. Savitz S, Caplan L. Vertebrobasilar disease. *N Engl J Med* 2005; **352**: 2618–26.

6. Amarenco P, Roullet E, Hommel M, Chaine P, Marteau R. Infarction in the territory of the medial branch of the posterior inferior cerebellar artery. *J Neurol Neurosurg Psychiatry* 1990; **53**: 731–5.

7. Lindsberg P, Mattle H. Therapy of basilar artery occlusion: a systematic analysis comparing intra-arterial and intravenous thrombolysis. *Stroke* 2006; **37**: 922–8.

8. Yu W, Binder D, Foster-Barber A, Malek R, Smith W, Higashida R. Endovascular embolectomy of acute basilar artery occlusion. *Neurology* 2003; **61**: 1421–3.

9. Schwarz S, Egelhof T, Schwab S, Hacke W. Basilar artery embolism: clinical syndrome and neuroradiologic patterns in patients without permanent occlusion of the basilar artery. *Neurology* 1997; **49**: 1346–52.

10. Osborn A. The posterior cerebral artery. In: *Diagnostic Cerebral Angiography*, 2nd edn. Philadelphia, PA: Lippincott Williams & Wilkins; 1999: 153–72.

11. Yamamoto Y, Georgiadis A, Chang H, Caplan L. Posterior cerebral artery territory infarcts in the New England Medical Center Posterior Circulation Registry. *Arch Neurol* 2000; **56**: 824–32.

12. Caplan LR. 'Top of the basilar' syndrome. *Neurology* 1980; **30**: 72–9.

13. Pessin M, Kwan E, Scott M, Hedges T. Occipital infarction with hemianopsia from carotid occlusive disease. *Stroke* 1989; **20**: 409–11.

14. Fisher C. Unusual vascular events in the territory of the posterior cerebral artery. *Can J Neurol Sci* 1986; **13**: 1–7.

15. Bogousslavsky J, Regli F, Uske A. Thalamic infarcts: clinical syndromes, etiology, and prognosis. *Neurology* 1988; **38**: 837–48.

16. Schmahmann J. Vascular syndromes of the thalamus. *Stroke* 2003; **34**: 2264–78.

17. Kameda W, Kawanami T, Kurita K, *et al.* Lateral and medial medullary infarction: a comparative analysis of 214 patients. *Stroke* 2004; **35**: 694–9.

18. Sacco R, Freddo L, Bello J, Odel J, Onesti S, Mohr J. Wallenberg's lateral medullary syndrome: clinical-magnetic resonance imaging correlations. *Arch Neurol* 1993; **50**: 609–14.

19. Brandt T, Kummer R, Muller–Kuppers M, Hacke W. Thrombolytic therapy of acute basilar artery occlusion: variables affecting recanalization and outcome. *Stroke* 1996; **27**: 875–81.

20. Ostrem J, Saver J, Alger J, *et al.* Acute basilar artery occlusion: diffusion–perfusion MRI characterization of tissue salvage in patients receiving intra-arterial stroke therapies. *Stroke* 2004; **35**: 30e–34e.

Further reading

Bogousslavsky J, Caplan L. *Stroke Syndromes*, 2nd edn. New York: Cambridge University Press; 2001.

Osborn A. *Diagnostic Neuroradiology*, 2nd edn. St Louis, MO: Mosby; 1994.

Tatu L, Moulin T, Bogousslavsky J, Duvernoy H. Arterial territories of human brain: brainstem and cerebellum. *Neurology* 1996; **47**: 1125–35.

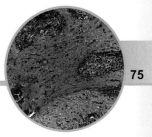

Chapter 5

Vasculopathies

Introduction

The most common arteriopathies responsible for stroke are large and small vessel atherosclerotic disease, which were discussed in the previous three chapters. However, a substantial percentage of strokes, particularly in younger patients, result from a variety of vasculopathies, in which different arterial wall layers develop pathology (**5.1**; *Table 5.1*). These causes fall into the 'Other determined etiology' (TOAST mechanism no. 4).[1]

This chapter surveys four of the most common vasculopathies: fibromuscular dysplasia (FMD), cervical artery dissection, vasculitis, and moyamoya.

Fibromuscular dysplasia

Definition

This systemic vasculopathy is caused by a proliferation of fibrous tissue (*fibroplasia*) in the smooth muscle layer of small- and medium-sized arteries. Smooth muscle cells are

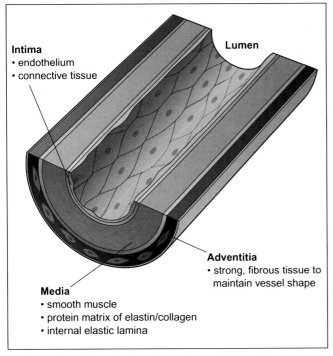

5.1 Vessel wall layers. The extracranial arterial walls layers are shown in this diagram. The intracranial arteries differ in their lack of the external elastic lamina and adventitia. Adapted with permission from Ross *et al.*[40]

Table 5.1 Common vasculopathies, by layer of the arterial wall involvement
Intima
• Atherosclerosis
• Cervical artery dissection
• Radiation arteriopathy
Media
• Cervical artery dissection
• Fibromuscular dysplasia
• Vasculitis; e.g., isolated CNS angiitis; temporal arteritis
Adventitia
• Cervical artery dissection
• Tumor invasion
Potential to involve multiple layers
• Moyamoya
• Sickle cell disease
• Cervical artery dissection
• Fibromuscular dysplasia
• Radiation arteriopathy
Adapted from Osborn.[4]

transformed into myofibroblasts, causing variable hyperplasia and thinning, with the destruction of elastic fibers. The pathology of FMD is entirely different from atherosclerosis (lipid accumulation, calcification, intimal plaque) and arteritis (inflammation and necrosis).[2,3] The etiology for FMD is unknown.

FMD most commonly affects medium-sized arteries, especially the renal and the cervical arteries.[3-5] The ICA is involved in 95% of all cervical cases, and in 60–85%

of cases the involvement of the ICA is bilateral. Usually, FMD spares the carotid bifurcation and occurs at the C1–C2 vertebral level, 3–4 cm distal to the ICA origin and may extend 0.5–7.0 cm (**5.2**). VA involvement is uncommon, but is usually opposite the C1 vertebral level, extending 1–2 cm. When complete angiographic studies are available, cerebrovascular and renal FMD coexists in up to 50% of patients.[5]

Pathogenesis of stroke

FMD is associated with numerous neurovascular disorders, including intracranial aneurysms[6] (**5.3**) and arteriovenous malformations (**5.4**). Stroke may result from various mechanisms:[5]

- *Artery-to-artery thromboembolism*: intravascular emboli presumably form within diverticular or pseudoaneurysmal sacs in the diseased arterial segment.
- *Cervical artery occlusive disease*:
  - arterial occlusion from extensive diverticuli causing stasis and subsequent occlusive disease, or dissection
  - hypoperfusion secondary to tight stenoses.
- *Dissection*: an estimated 10–20% of all spontaneous cervical arterial dissections are believed to be due to FMD, especially recurrent dissections and those affecting multiple vessels simultaneously.[7]
- *Subarachnoid hemorrhage* from rupture of intracranial aneurysms.

Diagnosis and differential diagnosis

FMD is a relatively common cause of stroke in young people. It should always be considered in younger stroke patients presenting with unexplained hypertension (which may be due to renal artery involvement (**5.5**)), cervical artery dissection, an incidental finding of a 'beading' pattern on non-invasive imaging of the ICA, and/or any cases where there is a family history of dissection, intracranial aneurysms, young stroke, and/or renal FMD.

Non-invasive computed tomography and magnetic resonance angiography (CTA and MRA) may detect FMD (**5.6**), but conventional angiography remains the gold standard for delineating the wide range of neurovascular lesions associated with FMD (**5.2–5.4**) and the angiographic subtypes of FMD (**5.7A**).[8]

True 'beading,' defined as alternating stenosis and aneurysmal dilatation of a cervical artery, is specific to FMD. However, the differential diagnosis for stenosis within the

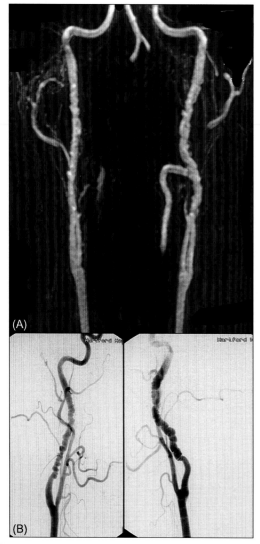

5.2 Fibromuscular dysplasia of the internal carotid arteries. This middle-aged patient with cervical bruits was found to have asymptomatic prominent bilateral ICA fibromuscular dysplasia on conventional angiography. A coronal MRA study of the ICAs (A); and on conventional angiography, common carotid injections, the ICAs are shown side-by-side (B). *Note*: extensive 'beading', regions of both stenosis and dilatation.

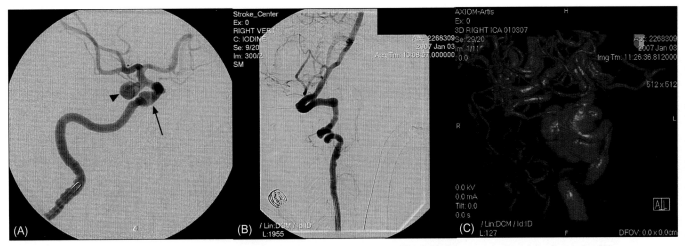

5.3 Intracranial aneurysms associated with fibromuscular dysplasia. A cervical ICA injection, conventional angiography (A), demonstrates a fusiform aneurysm (arrow) and saccular aneurysm (arrowhead) of the posterior communicating artery, with some typical beading of the cervical ICA at the level of the catheter tip. A second patient with fibromuscular dysplasia of the VA (B) had a cavernous ICA aneurysm, shown on a three-dimensional rendering of the conventional angiogram (C).

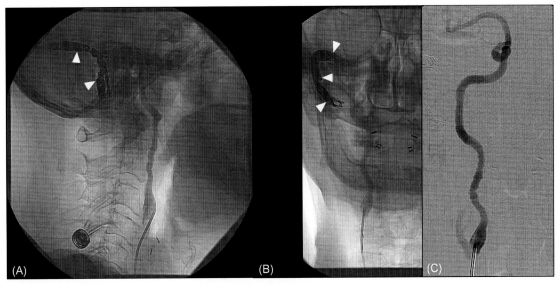

5.4 Dural arteriovenous fistula associated with fibromuscular dysplasia. This elderly woman presented with several years of right-sided tinnitus and a pulsatile bruit in the right mastoid region. A large dural arteriovenous fistula based in the right sigmoid sinus was treated with endovascular embolization to occlude the transverse sinus (arrowheads demarcate some of the coils used in this procedure). Fibromuscular dysplasia is readily appreciated in both the cervical ICA (A,B) and VA (C).

cervical and intracranial region is wide (*Table 5.2*).[4] A few arteriopathies closely resemble FMD (**5.7B**):

1 *Stationary arterial waves* are regular, evenly spaced transient constrictions during angiographic dye injections that are thought to be a physiologic response to local pressure from a catheter injection (**5.8**). They may occur quite distant from the injection site and will resolve spontaneously. The arterial wall diameter is unchanged in intervening segments.

2 *Catheter-induced vasospasm* typically occurs close to the catheter tip, with the potential for alternating stenosis with smooth or fusiform constrictions and dilation resembling FMD (**5.9**). Unlike FMD and vasospasm associated with subarachnoid hemorrhage, catheter-induced vasospasm is self-limited and rarely precipitates ischemic stroke.

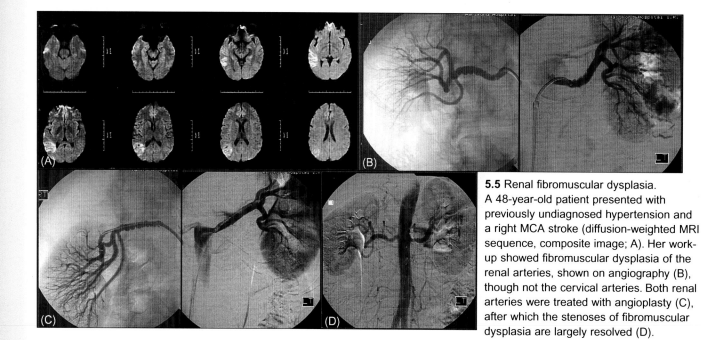

5.5 Renal fibromuscular dysplasia. A 48-year-old patient presented with previously undiagnosed hypertension and a right MCA stroke (diffusion-weighted MRI sequence, composite image; A). Her work-up showed fibromuscular dysplasia of the renal arteries, shown on angiography (B), though not the cervical arteries. Both renal arteries were treated with angioplasty (C), after which the stenoses of fibromuscular dysplasia are largely resolved (D).

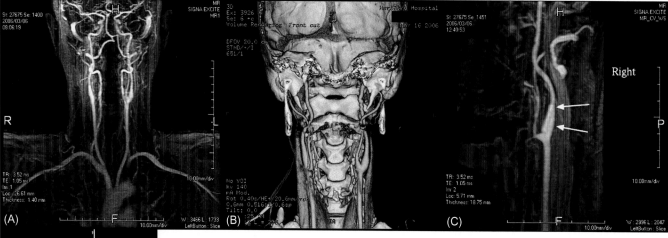

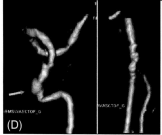

5.6 Cervical fibromuscular dysplasia on MRA and CT angiography. Coronal MRA (A) and CT angiography (B) show fibromuscular dysplasia of the ICA and VA, and a common associated finding, a dilated carotid bulb on MRA (arrows) (C). Focused segments of the cervical MRA show localized areas of dilatation and stenosis within the VA (D); on MRA, the 'waviness' of these segments resembles motion artifact.

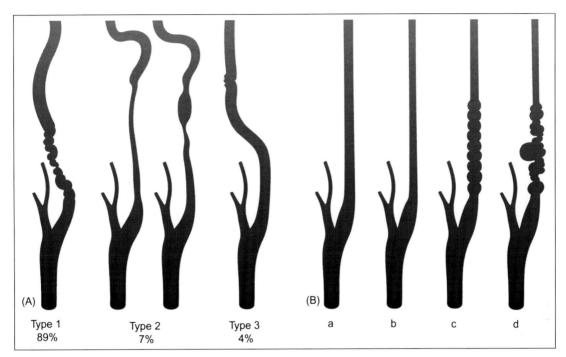

Type 1   Type 2   Type 3   a   b   c   d
89%   7%   4%

5.7 Cervical fibromuscular dysplasia. (A) The morphologic subtypes of cervical fibromuscular dysplasia. This schematic shows typical fibromuscular dysplasia of the ICA. Type 1 is the most common, but other forms with long areas of stenosis ('string signs') (type 2) and focal disease (type 3) have also been described. Adapted with permission from Osborn.[8] (B) Differential diagnosis for cervical fibromuscular dysplasia. The schematic shows a normal ICA (a), tubular (congenital) stenosis of the cervical ICA (b), stationary arterial waves (c), and fibromuscular dysplasia (d); see also *Table 5.2*. Adapted with permission from Osborn.[4]

Table 5.2 Differential diagnosis of segmental cervical and intracranial arterial narrowing

1. Atherosclerosis (B)
2. Cervical artery dissection (B,D)
3. Fibromuscular dysplasia (E,D)
4. Vasculitides (*Table 5.3*):
   (a) Takayasu's arteritis; giant cell arteritis (E)
   (b) Primary angiitis of the CNS (I)
5. Recanalizing embolism (I)
6. Radiation arteriopathy (E)
7. Moyamoya (I)
8. Tumor encasement
   (a) Meningioma, chordoma, pituitary adenoma (I)
   (b) Squamous cell carcinoma (E)
9. Iatrogenic mimics from cerebral angiography
   (a) Catheter-induced vasospasm (B)
   (b) Stationary arterial waves (E)
10. Ehlers–Danlos syndrome, type IV (E)
11. Neurofibromatosis (E)
12. Congenital hypoplasia/dysgenesis (E)

Predominant area of disease: I, intracranial; E, extracranial; B, both intracranial and extracranial involvement are common; D, commonly causes vessel dilatation as well as stenosis. Adapted from Osborn[4] and Zuber.[28]

3 Dissection alone may mimic focal forms of FMD (**5.7A**), and is best distinguished from FMD by natural history. Though stenosis secondary to dissection will often reopen or resolve, a stenosis due to FMD will not improve spontaneously (**5.10**).

Natural history and management

Minimal longitudinal data exist regarding the natural history of FMD as it relates to stroke risk. There is some documentation of gradual progression of FMD in cervical arterial disease. In a review of the literature, 23% (7 of 31) patients involved in serial cerebral angiographic studies developed mild to moderate degrees of progressive stenosis.[3] In patients followed up on medical (antiplatelet) treatment alone, several studies found a range of 0–4% annual risk of incident stroke or transient ischemic attack.[3]

No formal clinical trials exist regarding effective primary or secondary stroke prevention in patients with known cervical FMD. The standard for secondary stroke prevention is antiplatelet treatment, unless patients have high-grade hemodynamically significant stenosis and/or recurrent symptoms despite medical treatment. In this case, balloon

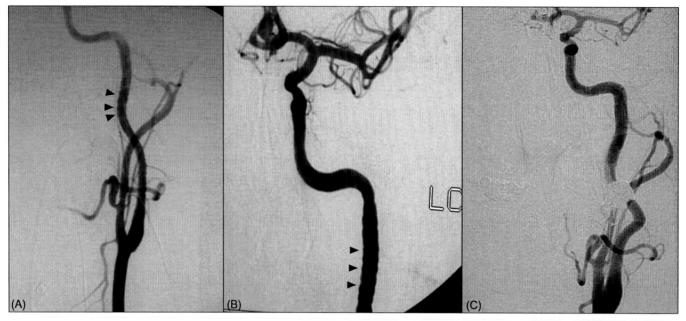

5.8 Stationary arterial waves. This common carotid injection shows stationary waves within the right cervical ICA (arrowheads) (A,B), which soon resolved following the dye injection (C).

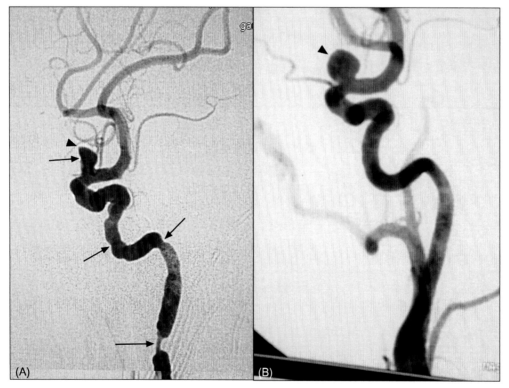

5.9 Catheter-induced vasospasm. Multifocal areas of stenosis (arrows) due to vasospasm of the parent ICA and an intracranial aneurysm (arrowhead) (A). The vasospasm entirely resolved on a later injection (B). In contrast with fibromuscular dysplasia, there are no areas of true arterial dilatation.

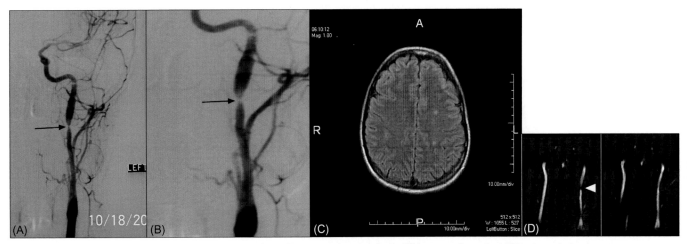

5.10 Focal cervical ICA stenosis: dissection versus focal fibromuscular dysplasia. This area of cervical ICA stenosis is shown on conventional angiography (arrows) (A,B). Small emboli to the left centrum semiovale occurred (FLAIR MRI sequence, C), causing mild right-sided deficits. The lesion is shown on coronal MRA sequences (D) the day after the angiographic study, showing the stenosis (arrowhead) (left), that had largely resolved on the repeat study 10 weeks later (right). The improvement in the stenosis is consistent with a local dissection rather than focal fibromuscular dysplasia.

angioplasty of cervical arteries may be pursued, and is technically straightforward (**case study 1**). The lesions of FMD may then be followed periodically with serial non-invasive studies, either MRA or CTA.

Cervical artery dissection

Definition

Dissection is a term derived from the Latin verb, *disseco*, indicating the separation of anatomic structures along natural lines by the tearing of the connective tissue framework. The resulting vascular lesion depends on which layer(s) of the artery are traumatized. Primary intimal tears, the most common lesion, result in subintimal hematomas. A false lumen develops, which may compromise the true lumen of the artery. More peripheral tears may involve either the media of the vessel wall, or the subadventitial space. The latter may result in aneurysmal dilatation of the vessel wall, which is called a dissecting aneurysm (**5.11**).[9–11]

Pathogenesis

The mobile components of the extracranial ICA and VA in the neck make them especially susceptible to dissection from head and neck trauma. Similar-sized vessels, such as the renal and coronary arteries, are much less prone to dissect, presumably because of less mobility. The ICA is usually injured within centimeters of the bulb, and the dissection frequently extends up to the entry point of the ICA at the

petrous bone into the skull (**5.12**). The VA is commonly injured at either the mid-cervical region at entry into the transverse foramen of the C6 vertebra or else at the most distal extracranial portion where the artery courses around the atlas to penetrate the dura mater (**5.13**).[10,11]

Several potential mechanisms for stroke are suggested by the common angiographic morphologies of ICA dissection (**5.11, 5.14**):[10,12]

- *Arterial occlusion.* An expanding arterial wall may compromise or occlude the true lumen of the artery, often resulting in a flame-shaped tapering of the cervical ICA (**5.15**). A low-flow state from severe stenosis (a 'string sign') (**5.16**) may also create local thrombosis via stasis, and/or borderzone infarction.
- *Artery-to-artery embolism:*
  - An intimal tear and medial hematoma may irritate the endothelium, precipitating the local formation of thrombi at the site of the tear, with exposure of subintimal thrombogenic elements within the bloodstream.[13,14] Multifocal small emboli may result (**5.17**).
  - Blood may dissect longitudinally and rupture back into the true lumen, injecting congealed hematoma to embolize upstream to the brain (**5.11, 5.12**).
  - The formation of thrombus may occur in mural pouches or the lumen of a *dissecting aneurysm* at a delayed interval, days to weeks following a dissection (**5.11, 5.12, 5.18; case study 2**).[15]

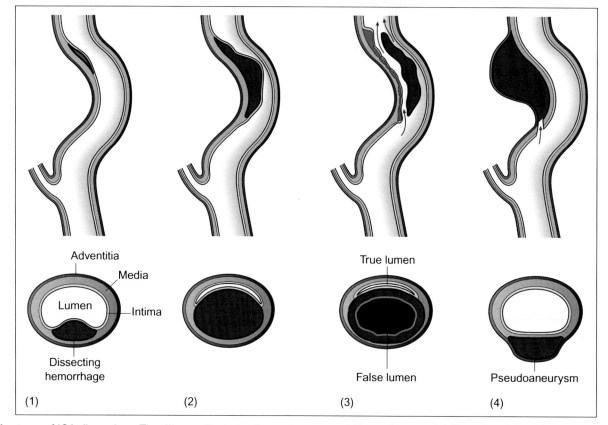

5.11 Anatomy of ICA dissections. The diagram illustrates the various presentations of an arterial dissection: (1) the false lumen partly occludes the artery, with a long string sign as the residual true lumen; (2) the false lumen largely occludes the artery, causing a tapered, proximal cervical ICA lesion; (3) the intramural hematoma of the false lumen ruptures back into the true lumen higher up within the cervical internal carotid artery; (4) aneurysmal dilatation, with an outward bowing of the healing vessel, a dissecting aneurysm is formed. Adapted with permission from Friedman *et al.*[9]

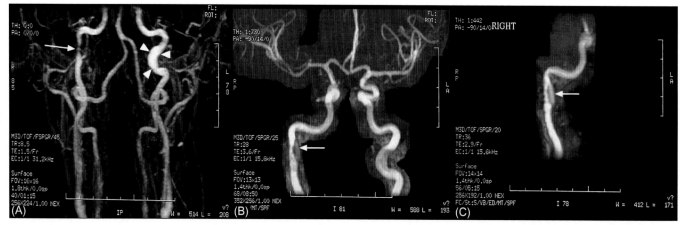

5.12 Bilateral cervical ICA dissections. A 40-year-old man presents with severe facial pain and right-sided Horner's syndrome. The initial coronal cervical MRA study (A) shows a high-grade high cervical ICA stenosis, just before the level of the petrous bone (arrow), and the contralateral side has a chronic dissecting aneurysm at a similar level (arrowheads). An isolated view of the anterior circulation raises the possibility of a false lumen adjacent (medial) to the true lumen (arrow) (B), better appreciated when the cervical right ICA is isolated (C).

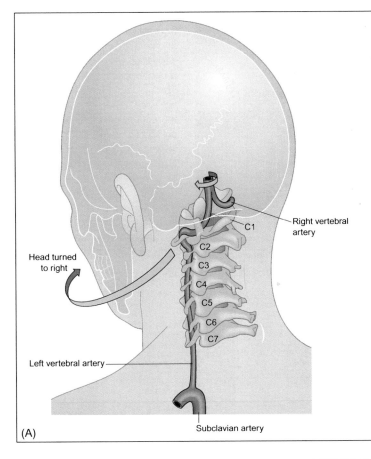

(A)

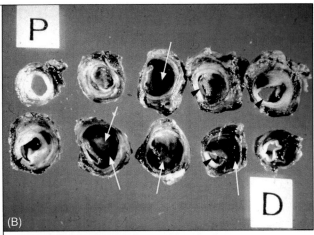

(B)

5.13 VA dissection: anatomy and gross pathology. (A) The VA is commonly dissected at two areas: (1) around the transverse foramina from C4 to C6, due to contact and pressure from osteophytes and from local skeletal muscles and fasciobends in this proximal segment; and (2) from stretch injury between the C1 and C2 vertebral transverse foraminae, when the head is sharply turned. Adapted with permission from Krueger et al.[41] (B) Serial transverse sections of a dissected vertebral artery are shown from proximal (P, upper left) to distal (D, lower right). Note the intramural hematoma (arrows) and varying degrees of occlusion of the true lumen (arrowheads). Pathology courtesy of Louis Caplan, MD.

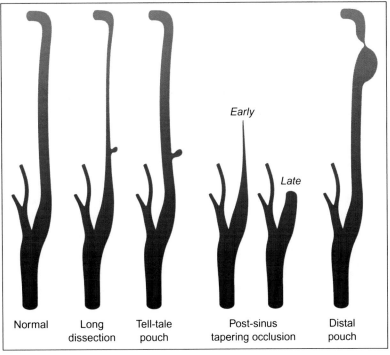

5.14 Common angiographic features of internal carotid artery dissection. Adapted from Fisher et al.[42]

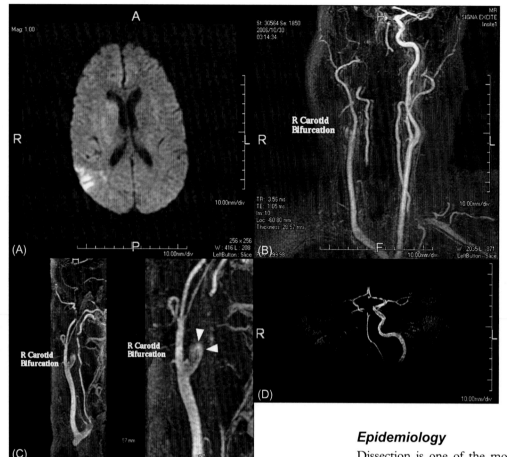

5.15 Right ICA occlusion from dissection. A right MCA stroke, diffusion-weighted MRI sequence (A), resulting from a right cervical ICA occlusion. The coronal MRA shows an absence of flow signal through the entire right cervical ICA portion (B), while focused views of the right neck show a bullet-shaped tapering of the occluded artery (arrowheads) (C). Intracranial MRA shows a healthy proximal right MCA, supplied via the anterior and posterior communicating arteries (D).

• *Aortic dissection.* This more proximal arterial dissection normally presents with a distinct history and symptoms, such as blunt trauma to the chest, chest pain, asymmetric blood pressures, and cardiovascular instability, not typical for dissection of the cervical arteries alone. However, cerebral thromboembolism and cervical artery occlusion may occur as a complication of aortic dissection (**5.19**).

Most cervical artery dissections are spontaneous. A variety of colorful anecdotes of physical activities and head–neck trauma have been reported to cause cervical artery dissections.[7,10] An underlying arteriopathy is not usually identified, though several heritable connective tissue disorders have been associated with dissection.[7,16–18] A developmental syndrome of neural crest cells, the familial syndrome of arterial dissections with lentiginosis, has been linked to cervical artery dissection.[16] Connective tissue and other genetic disorders should be considered when multiple or recurrent dissections occur, or a family history of young stroke or dissection exist.

Epidemiology

Dissection is one of the most common causes of thrombus formation in cervical arteries. It is probably the second leading cause of cervical ICA occlusion, though well behind atherosclerotic disease. The mean age at presentation with cervical artery dissection is only 45 years, perhaps relating to the elasticity and extensibility of these arteries in younger patients.[7,16] Cervical artery dissection in patients >65 years of age is rare and is generally caused by significant head–neck trauma.

Clinical syndrome

The triad of facial, head, or neck pain, a Horner's syndrome, and delayed cerebral or retinal ischemia are strong evidence for cervical artery dissection. In the absence of stroke, dissection may be misdiagnosed as a common or complicated migraine.[19] A partial Horner's syndrome (miosis and ptosis without anhidrosis) results from aneurysmal compression of the oculosympathetic chain in ICA dissection (**5.20**). In VA dissection, Horner's syndrome may result from infarction of the lateral medulla. The presence of cerebrovascular symptoms in a person of younger age with any headache or neck pain should prompt a diagnostic evaluation for cervical artery dissection.

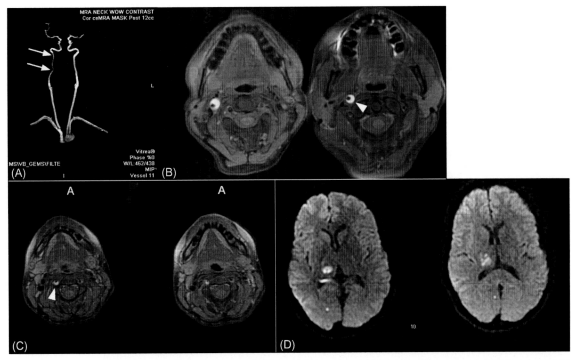

5.16 The 'halo sign' of cervical artery dissection. A 53-year-old woman presented with a severe right hemicranial headache, but a normal examination and no history or imaging findings of stroke. The MRA studies isolating the bilateral ICAs (A) show a smooth tapering toward a 'string sign' (arrows) through much of the mid-upper cervical extent of the right ICA. A classic 'halo sign' is prominently observed on adjacent transaxial T1 fat-saturated sequences (arrowhead) (B). A 35-year-old woman presented with cervical pain while jogging, and subsequently developed mild gait ataxia and left hemisensory symptoms. The T1 fat-saturated sequence (C) documented a 'halo sign' of the right cervical VA (arrowhead). The diffusion-weighted MRI sequences identify an embolic right PCA-territory stroke, involving predominantly the thalamus (D).

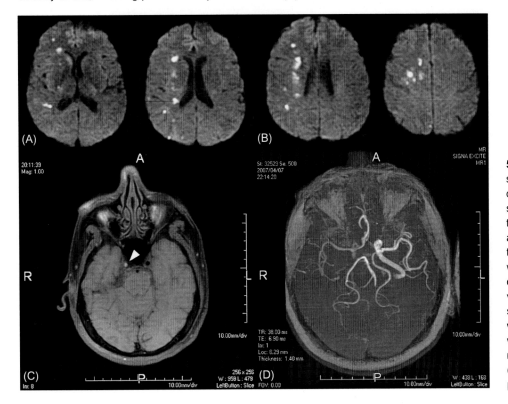

5.17 Right hemispheric embolic shower from internal carotid artery dissection. Diffusion-weighted sequences show multifocal emboli to the MCA–MCA borderzone on adjacent diffusion-weighted MRI transaxial series (A,B). The source was cervical ICA occlusion due to dissection, with absence of flow void on the transaxial T1-weighted segment (arrowhead) compared with the left distal ICA (C). There was no apparent filling of the distal right ICA on the intracranial MRA (D), with diminished flow into the proximal right MCA.

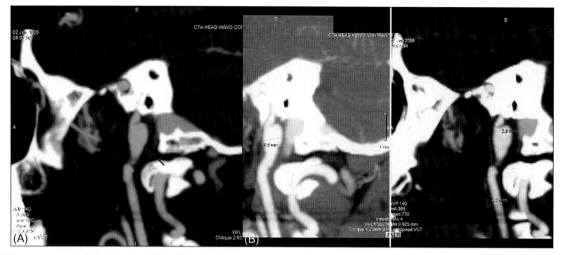

5.18 Dissecting aneurysm of the cervical ICA. CT angiography, sagittal view (A), in a patient with cervical fibromuscular dysplasia demonstrates this aneurysmal dilatation close to the skull base (arrows). The lesion is measured at the maximum diameter of the aneurysmal widening (B, left), and is roughly three times the lumen of the ICA just above the lesion (B, right).

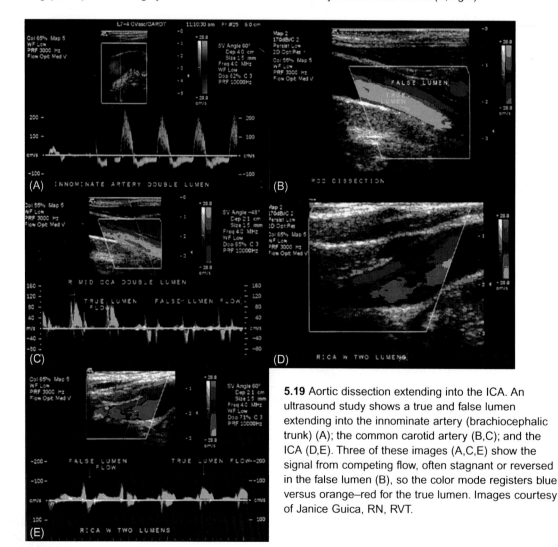

5.19 Aortic dissection extending into the ICA. An ultrasound study shows a true and false lumen extending into the innominate artery (brachiocephalic trunk) (A); the common carotid artery (B,C); and the ICA (D,E). Three of these images (A,C,E) show the signal from competing flow, often stagnant or reversed in the false lumen (B), so the color mode registers blue versus orange–red for the true lumen. Images courtesy of Janice Guica, RN, RVT.

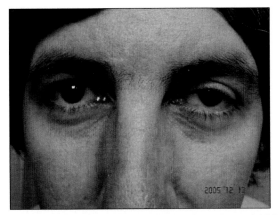

5.20 Horner's syndrome associated with a traumatic left ICA dissection in a 43-year-old man. Note ptosis and (less evident) miosis OS. Image courtesy of Robert Lesser, MD.

Diagnosis

Non-invasive imaging, particularly transaxial fat-saturated T1-weighted MRI, has supplanted angiography as the urgent diagnostic modality of choice. The pathognomonic 'halo sign' of intramural hematoma is often well-visualized as a hyperintense signal early in the course of ICA dissection (**5.16B**). It is often more difficult to visualize in VA dissections, due to their smaller lumen size (**5.16C**). Ultrasound is not as useful in diagnosis; this is because most cervical artery dissections occur higher in the neck than can be readily accessed with an external ultrasound probe (**5.19**).

Natural history

The natural history of stroke due to cervical artery dissection is reasonably benign. In a large prospective series of patients with a first cervical artery dissection ($n = 459$), there were a total of only four recurrent dissections (0.9%) and four recurrent ischemic strokes (two attributable to the initial dissection, and two from recurrent dissections) in almost 3 years of follow-up.[20] Dissections do not typically recur in the same vessel, perhaps due to the local healing process.

Management
Secondary stroke prevention

The most efficacious antithrombotic regimen to best prevent recurrent stroke following cervical artery dissection remains unresolved, but may be tailored toward the individual lesion. Anticoagulation with warfarin could presumably prevent recurrent thromboemboli from a highly stenotic or occluded extracranial cervical artery. Concern about the use of anticoagulation relates to the rare, life-threatening

potential complication of subarachnoid hemorrhage that may occur whenever a cervical artery dissection extends intracranially. Anticoagulation has not been documented to cause propagation or expansion of an intramural hematoma. The consensus approach to treatment in most patients following acute extracranial dissection is anticoagulation for 2–3 months, and then conversion to antiplatelet treatment. Follow-up MRA or CTA at 3 months is used to gauge the artery's recanalization and any luminal irregularities (**5.10D**).

Acute interventions

Some data suggest that intravenous thrombolysis does not pose a specific risk to patients with acute cervical artery dissection. In case series, there has been no apparent risk of worsening the primary intramural hematoma, nor additional risk of intracranial extension or aneurysmal dilatation.[21,22] Endovascular interventions for acute dissection are technically challenging due to the fluctuating nature of the lesion, the difficulty in differentiating the true from the false lumen, and the risk of rupturing through the arterial wall. In very high-risk situations where there is a compromise of multiple cervical arteries, interventional procedures can be considered, e.g., angioplasty, stenting (**case study 3**),[18,23] neurosurgical trapping, vascular bypass, treatment of an intracranial thromboembolic lesion caused by an extracranial dissection (**case study 4**), or endovascular coiling with sacrifice of a cervical artery.

Vasculitis

Definition

Systemic vasculitis includes a group of disorders where inflammation and destruction (necrosis) of the vessel wall is the primary event.[24-29] Both primary (idiopathic) and secondary (those associated with infectious and non-infectious inflammatory diseases) vasculitides (**5.21**) can cause cerebral vasculitis (*Table 5.3*). This section will briefly review giant cell arteritis (GCA) and primary central nervous system (CNS) angiitis.

Clinical presentation and epidemiology

A common cause of headache in patients >50 years of age, GCA is the most common vasculitis to cause cerebrovascular symptoms. It is a systemic arteritis of medium- and large-caliber arteries anywhere in the body, with a predilection for the extracranial cervical arteries. The diagnosis should be considered in patients with a variety of symptoms:

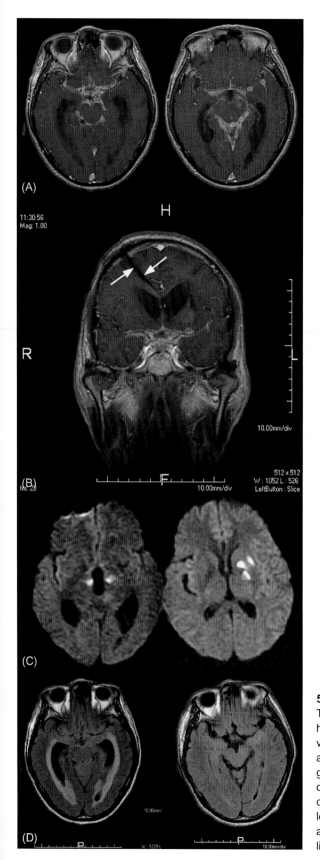

headache, visual loss and/or diplopia, pain on continuous chewing (jaw claudication) or swallowing, fever, and other constitutional symptoms (anorexia, weight loss, malaise), and the stiffness of polymyalgia rheumatica, a commonly associated syndrome.[29] Serologic markers of inflammation, erythrocyte sedimentation rate and C-reactive protein, are typically elevated. Physical signs of GCA include swollen,

---

Table 5.3 Types of vasculitis

1. *Primary CNS vasculitis* (primary angiitis of the CNS, granulomatous angiitis)
2. *Systemic vasculitis with CNS involvement*
   (a) Systemic necrotizing vasculitis: polyarteritis nodosa; Churg–Strauss syndrome
   (b) Wegener's granulomatosis
   (c) Behçet's disease
   (d) Giant cell arteritis: Takayasu's arteritis; giant cell arteritis
3. *Systemic diseases with secondary CNS angiitis, or vasculopathy*
   (a) Scleroderma
   (b) Rheumatoid disease
   (c) Sjögren's syndrome
   (d) Antiphospholipid antibody syndrome
   (e) Systemic lupus erythematosus
4. *CNS disorders with secondary vasculitis*
   (a) Meningitis: pyogenic, tuberculous, fungal, parasitic, syphilitic
   (b) Septic emboli
   (c) Non-granulomatous inflammations: neurosarcoidosis

CNS, central nervous system.
Adapted from Osborn[4] and Zuber.[28]

5.21 Tuberculous meningitis causing arachnoiditis and secondary vasculitis. This patient developed an encephalopathy due to meningitis, obstructive hydrocephalus, and deep cerebral infarcts caused by proximal intracranial vasculitis. The first MRI scan shows extensive basal meningitis and arachnoiditis on adjacent transaxial cuts (A) and coronal (B) T1WI with gadolinium, lining the region of the circle of Willis. The linear dark structure on this coronal sequence is an intraventricular catheter (arrows). Infarcts developed in the cerebellar vermis, as well as the bilateral rostral thalami (C, left), and 3 weeks later, in the left lenticulostriate territory (C, right). Following an antitubercular medical regimen, the basal meningitis, with inflammation lining the lateral ventricles and hydrocephalus (D, left), resolved (D, right).

painful superficial temporal arteries, scalp necrosis and tenderness, ischemic optic neuropathy, and posterior circulation ischemic stroke. Longitudinal epidemiological studies note an incidence of 17.0 persons per 100 000 population >50 years of age.[29]

Primary (or isolated) CNS angiitis has a wide range of presenting symptoms, so it is frequently included in the differential diagnosis of neurovascular syndromes. CNS angiitis can cause seizures, intracerebral hemorrhage, acute ischemic stroke, headaches, and psychiatric symptoms. Untreated, the disease often results in recurrent brain injury and significant morbidity and mortality. This localized disease of small- and medium-sized intracranial arteries is decidedly rare, with an incidence estimated at <1:2 000 000.[28]

Pathogenesis and diagnosis

The diagnosis of GCA is typically made by a biopsy of the superficial temporal arteries (**5.22**). The involvement of the extracranial external carotid and vertebral arteries is apparently explained by the disease's predilection for arteries with a high elastic content in the arterial media and adventitia.[27,29] The four vessels most commonly affected in GCA are the superficial temporal, ophthalmic, posterior ciliary, and vertebral arteries. Arteritic ischemic optic neuropathy causing blindness, the most common severe morbidity from GCA, is due to local involvement of the posterior ciliary arteries. Visual loss can rapidly evolve in both eyes within days.[29] The uncommon association of GCA with ischemic stroke is almost always from local thromboembolic disease developing in vertebral arteries. The local arteritic disease typically extends only 5 mm above the dural perforation of the vertebral arteries, where the external elastic lamina ends.[27]

The diagnosis of primary CNS angiitis is also dependent on tissue examination, though it is considered in cases where there are multifocal intracranial lesions, without the presence of a systemic vasculitis. The absence of other organ involvement and normal serologic tests point to a diagnosis of primary CNS angiitis. Neuroimaging (CT and MRI findings) can delineate the extent of CNS involvement, but there are no findings specific to vasculitis. While the cerebrospinal fluid (CSF) is usually abnormal with, at minimum, a lymphocytic pleocytosis and/or elevated protein, the angiographic picture is non-specific and can be seen with other conditions causing vasoconstriction (**5.23**) or vasospasm, or the commonly seen changes due to atherosclerosis (**5.24**).[30] Brain and/or meningeal biopsy are usually required for a definitive diagnosis, documenting

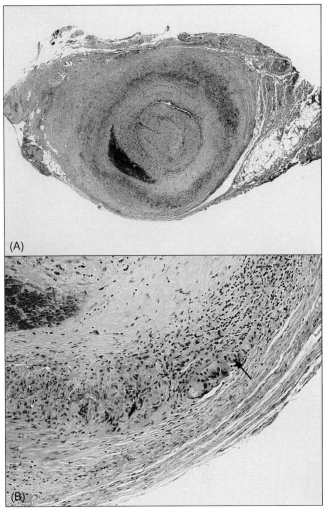

5.22 Temporal arteritis, pathology. Complete occlusion of the superficial temporal artery, due to an inflammatory process within the artery's walls (A) (hematoxylin and eosin stain, 40×). The outer layers of the wall, at higher power, demonstrate giant mononuclear (Langherhans) cells (arrow), diagnostic for temporal arteritis (hematoxylin and eosin, 100×) (B). Pathology courtesy of Robert Schmidt MD, PhD.

granulomatous involvement of the small- and medium-sized intracranial arteries (**5.25**). Given that the treatment is long-term, using immunomodulatory agents, biopsy confirmation of the diagnosis is a critical step in management.

Management

Urgent treatment of GCA with intravenous steroids is indicated when visual loss develops, often to protect the contralateral eye (if the symptomatic eye does not improve). A transition to a long-term tapering regimen with prednisone in much higher

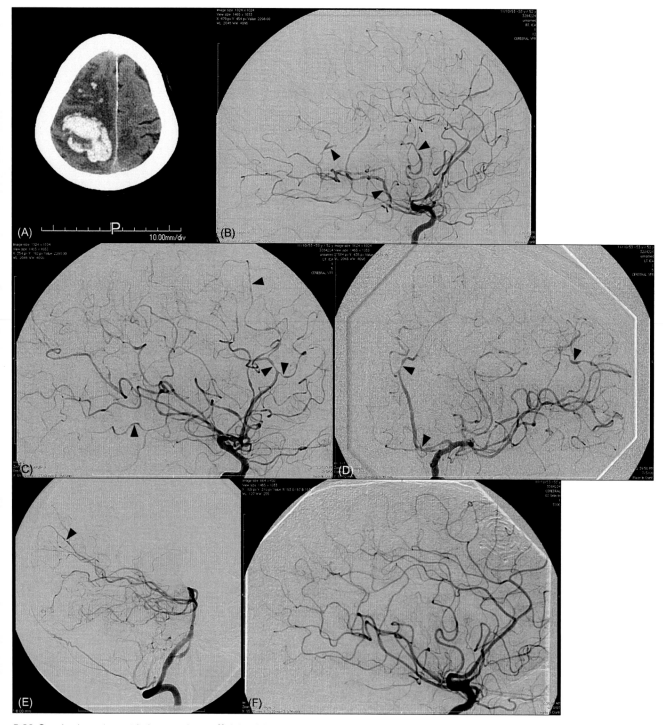

5.23 Cerebral vasoconstriction syndrome.[30] A healthy 50-year-old woman presented with headache, confusion, and left-sided deficits from a right lobar parietal hemorrhage (A). Initial conventional angiography shows right ICA injection, lateral view (B); left ICA injections, lateral (C) and oblique (D) views; and left VA injection (E). Note multifocal stenoses and irregularities, more prominent in the anterior than the posterior circulation (arrowheads). The working initial diagnosis was primary CNS angiitis, and the patient was first treated with prednisone and cyclophosphamide. However, the admission cerebrospinal fluid study was unremarkable, as was the follow-up angiography, obtained 9 months after the first. This second study showed complete resolution of the arteriopathy on a right ICA injection, oblique view (F).

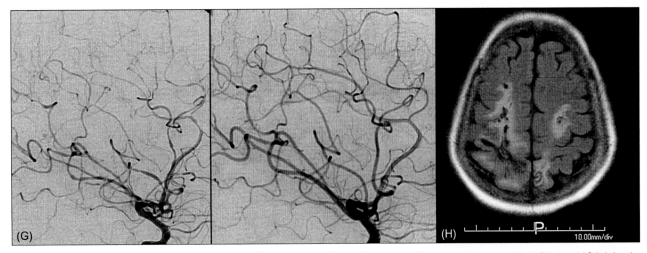

(G) (H) 10.00mm/div

5.23 (*continued*) Cerebral vasoconstriction syndrome.[30] The final angiographic images juxtapose comparable left lateral ICA injections from the initial study (G, left) and the follow-up study (G, right). Note the markedly improved caliber of most distal arterial segments. Repeat MRI scan, FLAIR sequence, 5 months later, shows the previous right lobar parietal hemorrhage (A) as well as small-vessel intracranial disease (H). At 14 months after the presentation, the patient was doing well, with predominantly left arm paresis and mild left-sided neglect.

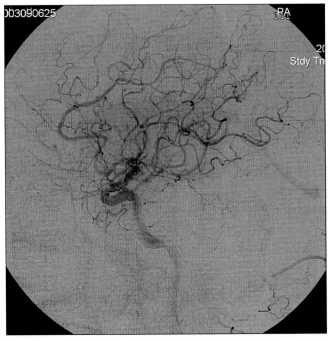

5.24 Intracranial atherosclerosis. An 80-year-old man was treated for acute ischemic stroke with intra-arterial thrombolysis. On this post-treatment lateral view, ICA injection, late arterial phase, the hemispheric arteries are shown to demonstrate that tortuosity, stenosis, and large vessel irregularities are quite common in atherosclerosis, and may mimic vasculitis.

doses than are employed for polymyalgia rheumatica is then indicated. The patient's clinical syndrome and erythrocyte sedimentation rate are followed over time. The main non-steroid agent that has been studied is azathioprine.[29]

Because of its rarity, the best treatment for biopsy-proven primary CNS angiitis is unresolved. Steroids and other immunomodulatory agents, in particular cyclophospha-mide, often in combination, are considered the standard to prevent disease progression; however, no controlled clinical trials of this rare disorder have been undertaken. Disease activity may be followed by the clinical course as well as with serial examinations of cerebrospinal fluid and/or serial conventional angiographic studies.[28]

Moyamoya

Definition and pathogenesis

Moyamoya means 'puff of smoke' and refers to the classic angiographic picture seen in this syndrome. This non-inflammatory occlusive intracranial arteriopathy results in progressive bilateral obliteration of the major arteries of the anterior circulation, the ICA, ACA, and MCA. After initial segmental narrowing of the distal ICAs (**5.26**), the first moyamoya vasculature develops, with a telangiectatic network of collaterals deep in the hemispheres (**case study 5**).[31–33]

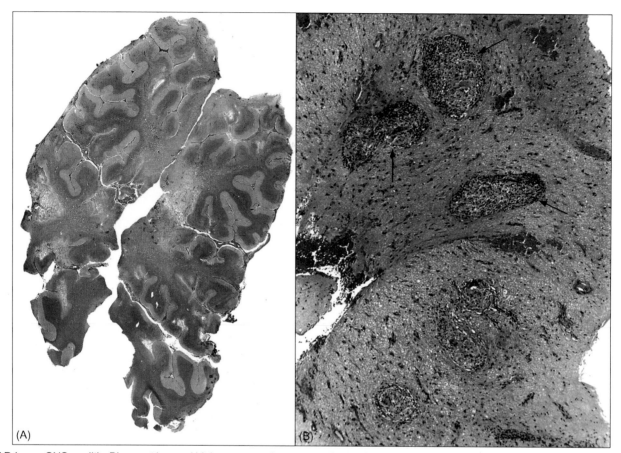

5.25 Primary CNS angiitis. Biopsy at low and higher powers show areas of pallor from ischemia within a sample of cerebellar tissue, including granular layers (A) (hematoxylin and eosin stain, 40×), as well as multiple granulomas (arrows), localized to the Virchow Robbins spaces and (not shown) within arteriolar walls (B) (hematoxylin and eosin, 100×). Pathology courtesy of Robert Schmidt MD, PhD.

Finally, regression of the moyamoya vessels occurs, with concurrent growth of meningeal–pial collaterals from the external carotid artery to supply much of the cerebral hemispheres.[32] The basic underlying pathophysiology of moyamoya disease is unknown.

Epidemiology

The moyamoya syndrome can be primary (**moyamoya disease**) (**5.26**) or secondary to a variety of underlying diseases that may be due to infectious, inflammatory, vasculopathic, genetic, or hematologic/prothrombotic disorders (**moyamoya syndrome**).[32] About 10% of cases are unilateral and 10% genetic, occurring most frequently in Japanese and other Asian populations.

Natural history and management

The natural history is somewhat different for Asians, who more often have moyamoya disease (**5.26**), and Caucasians, who are more likely to have a moyamoya syndrome. Asian children present with ischemic stroke, while hemorrhagic stroke becomes more common in adulthood. In Caucasians, ischemic stroke is most common at any age.[34,35]

Moyamoya is a progressive disorder with unfavorable outcomes predominating. The progression of the disease as documented by angiography is much more aggressive in childhood than in adulthood, but the prognosis for functional status and life expectancy is poor in adults due to recurrent hemorrhages.[36]

Moyamoya disease is generally treated by a surgical revascularization procedure. The two major types of revascularizations are a superficial temporal artery-to-MCA direct bypass provided that an acceptable cortical branch of the MCA exists for anastomosis and an indirect revascularization procedure known as encephaloduroarteriosynangiosis.[32,37–39] In the latter case, a bone window is made to enable the surgeon to directly

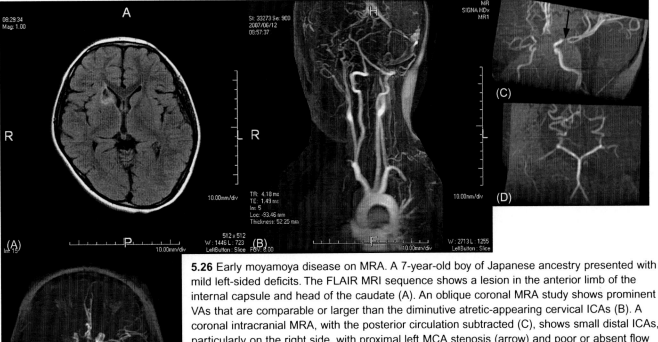

5.26 Early moyamoya disease on MRA. A 7-year-old boy of Japanese ancestry presented with mild left-sided deficits. The FLAIR MRI sequence shows a lesion in the anterior limb of the internal capsule and head of the caudate (A). An oblique coronal MRA study shows prominent VAs that are comparable or larger than the diminutive atretic-appearing cervical ICAs (B). A coronal intracranial MRA, with the posterior circulation subtracted (C), shows small distal ICAs, particularly on the right side, with proximal left MCA stenosis (arrow) and poor or absent flow through the A1 segments bilaterally and the right M1 segment. By contrast, the A2 and more distal ACA segments have a strong signal. A focused view of the posterior circulation (D) shows prominent PCA anatomy, also seen on a transaxial intracranial MRA study (E). This last study suggests minimal or poor perfusion of MCA branches throughout the right hemisphere, with possible collateral supply from a lateral PCA branch (arrowhead) and/or extracranial leptomeningeal supply. This MRA shows occlusive obliteration of the distal ICAs and proximal ACA and MCA segments typical of early moyamoya disease. A conventional angiogram would be needed to completely delineate the vasculature, but the telangiectatic moyamoya pattern may not yet have developed. This patient's presenting stroke reflects the severe vasculopathy within the right A1 and M1 segments.

suture the superficial temporal artery to the pia matter. In successful cases, extracranial-to-intracranial angiogenesis (new collateral vessels) develop over several months that augment hemispheric blood flow (**case study 5**). Combined direct and indirect revascularizations are also feasible, but controlled clinical trials and long-term follow-up documenting benefits in terms of functional status and cognitive improvement are lacking.[36]

Case studies

Case study 1. Angioplasty of cervical fibromuscular dysplasia

The bilateral, severe FMD of the cervical ICA shown (**CS 1.1**) was measured: right (A) and left (B), and then both sides were treated with angioplasty. The images show progressive dilatation of the left cervical disease (C),

to 4 mmHg balloon pressure (left) and, later, 5 mmHg (right).

Comments

The balloon pressure for progressive arterial dilation during angioplasty of FMD is only 5–6 atmospheres, versus 15–20 for atherosclerotic stenosis.[5] Primary angioplasty alone is quite effective for resolving focal stenoses and may be repeated, if necessary. The risk of employing endovascular stents for the treatment of FMD-related stenosis is unknown, but overgrowth of an *in situ* stent by intimal or medial fibroplasia is theoretically possible.

Case study 2. Vertebral artery dissecting aneurysm treated with stenting

A middle-aged man presented with a right lateral medullary infarction (not shown) associated with this traumatic right

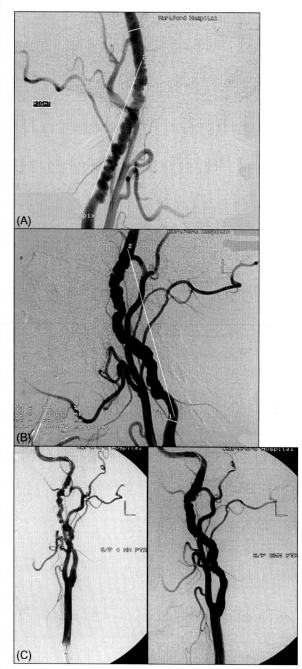

CS 1.1

VA dissection. A distal right VA dissection with a small false lumen is shown on conventional angiography (**CS 2.1A**) and reconstructed three-dimensional images (B,C). The true lumen constitutes only a string sign (arrows) (A).

This lesion did not improve over the initial 3 months, prompting a decision to treat with angioplasty and stenting of the artery to re-establish the lumen and prevent recurrent

thromboembolization. The final image (D) is a CT angiogram in which the proximal and distal stent margins appear as white markers. The right PICA is seen behind its parent VA. (*Note*: the left and right sides are reversed on this CTA.)

Case study 3. Bilateral internal carotid artery dissections with unilateral angioplasty and stenting

A 36-year-old woman suffered bilateral severe ICA dissections while horseback-riding (**CS 3.1**). The initial cervical MRA shows flame-shaped tapering of both cervical ICAs, with possible occlusions (A). A borderzone stroke, shown on the diffusion-weighted MRI sequence (B), caused mild left hemiparesis, predominantly affecting the hand.

Conventional cerebral angiography (**CS 3.2**) showed a tapered left ICA that appears completely occluded (arrows), with the catheter tip at the beginning of the tapering (A), as well as a long severe string sign of the right ICA, with reconstitution at the level of the petrous bone (arrow) (B).

Two stents were placed (**CS 3.3**) in order to expand the true lumen, as shown on the unsubtracted (A, left) and subtracted (A, right) lateral views, with excellent result. A post-stent ICA injection (B) shows excellent filling of the right hemisphere, including the right fetal posterior cerebral artery (PCA) and also, via the anterior communicating artery, the left ACA. The patient remained without further symptoms on subcutaneous enoxaparin and clopidogrel.

A follow-up MRA study (**CS 3.4**) 3 months from the initial dissections showed apparent recanalization in the left cervical ICA (A, left; reconstructed coronal image; note the artifact produced in the region of the right ICA stents (arrowheads). An intracranial MRA (A, right) shows normal ICA siphon flow bilaterally. The final infarct is shown on T2WI at 3 months (B); the patient had only mild slowing of fine finger movements in the left hand, and anticoagulation was discontinued.

Comments

For a number of reasons a decision was made to treat the right ICA lesion first (versus the left ICA) with angioplasty and stenting. The right carotid dissection appeared more accessible, with a more viable lumen. The periprocedural risk might be lower because the right ICA supplies the non-dominant hemisphere. The right hemispheric flow demonstrated (with stroke) a more critical hemodynamic insufficiency than the left hemisphere. Finally, the right ICA also supplied the fetal PCA, putting a larger area of the brain at risk for stroke.

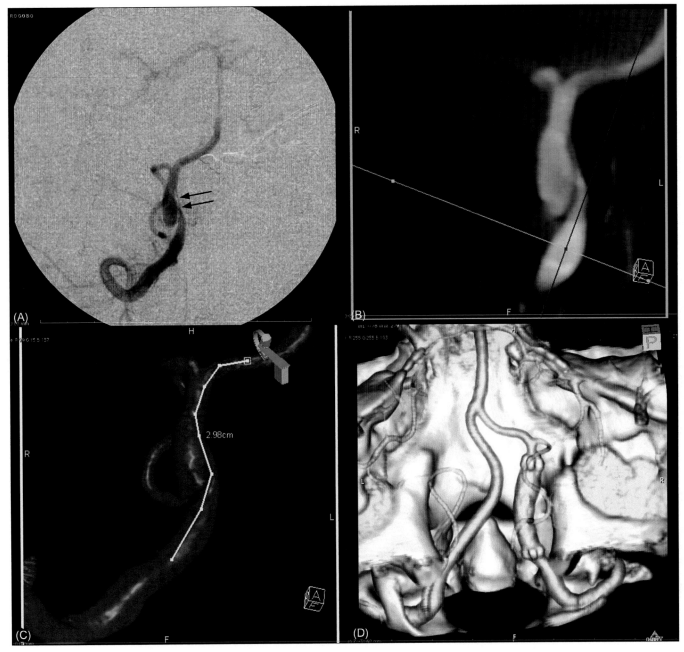

CS 2.1

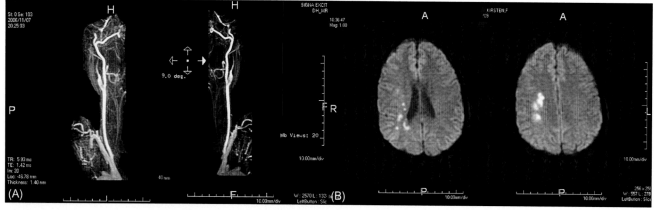

CS 3.1

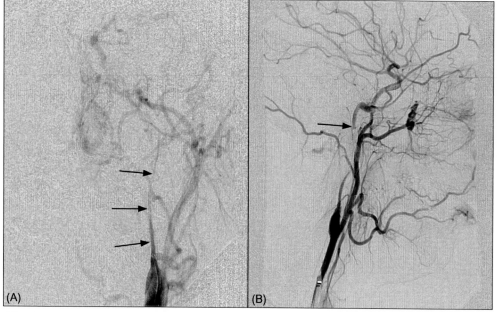

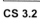

CS 3.2

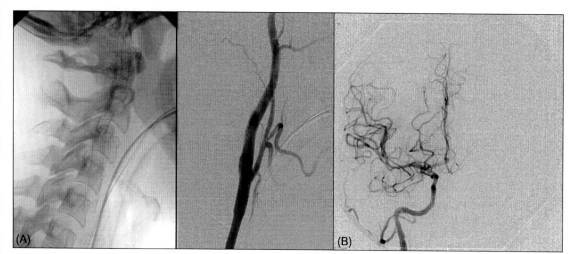

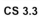

CS 3.3

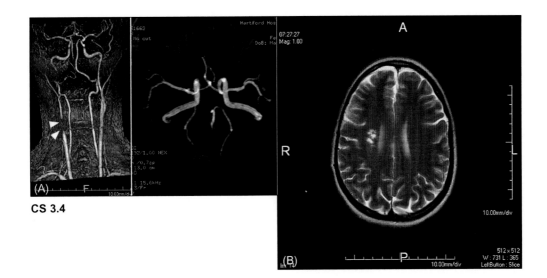

CS 3.4

Case study 4. Urgent stenting of middle cerebral artery occlusion due to internal carotid artery dissection

The patient was treated for acute subcortical right MCA ischemic stroke, which had been caused by right cervical ICA dissection embolizing into the MCA territory; this was preceded by several hours of monocular right-sided blindness, due to previous embolism in the central retinal artery (not shown). The diffusion-weighted MRI sequence 1 day later is shown (**CS 4.1**).

Conventional angiography performed on admission shows a flame-shaped right ICA dissection (**CS 4.2**). On common carotid artery injection, the lesion appears occlusive (A, left), but an ICA injection shows a string sign (arrowheads) with some reconstitution of the lumen before the petrous level (A, right; arrow). Treatment of the ICA terminus thrombus extending into the MCA with intra-arterial thrombolysis was unsuccessful. The MCA lesion is shown before (B, left) and immediately after (B, right) infusion of 12 mg intra-arterial tissue plasminogen activator; however, this recanalization was only transient.

Endovascular angioplasty and stenting of the MCA was pursued next. Two Neuroform™ stents were placed in a bifurcative fashion into the superior and inferior divisions. The initial stent (3 mm × 20 mm, width by length), placed within the superior branch, is shown on a local injection, anteroposterior view (C, left), and then, local injection with a guidewire into the inferior branch before the second stent (C, right).

Next, two stents were placed more proximally within the petrous ICA lesion with initial restoration of antegrade flow through the cervical ICA (not shown). However, on a follow-up CTA study 2 months later (**CS 4.3**), a transaxial cut shows the right cervical ICA stent (arrowhead) (A) has become occluded, in contrast to the hyperdense normal flow signal within the contralateral ICA (arrow). The intracranial MCA stents on non-contrast CT scans create local artifacts (B). Intact flow through the stents is evident on the source images of the MRA study; compare the right and left M1 and M2 segments coursing into the Sylvian fissures (C).

Comments

This patient had a complex tandem lesion, with a typical cervical ICA dissection that embolized to both the lenticulostriate arteries and the central retinal artery (e.g., see also Chapter 3, **case study 1**). The lesion with the highest risk, the right distal ICA and M1 thrombus, was treated with stenting after intra-arterial thrombolysis failed. Given the subsequent thrombosis in the cervical ICA stenting,

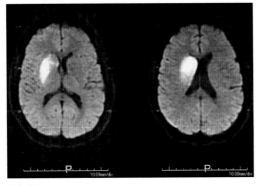

CS 4.1

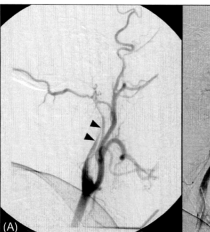
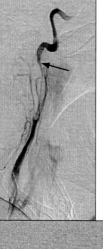

collateral flow from the anterior communicating artery likely played a major part in limiting the eventual size of the right hemispheric infarct.

At 2 years post-stroke, the patient's sole deficit is monocular blindness from the retinal lesion, with no residual deficits associated with the cerebral lesion. The old right MCA territory stroke, with *ex vacuo* enlargement of the frontal horn of the lateral ventricle, is shown (**CS 4.4**).

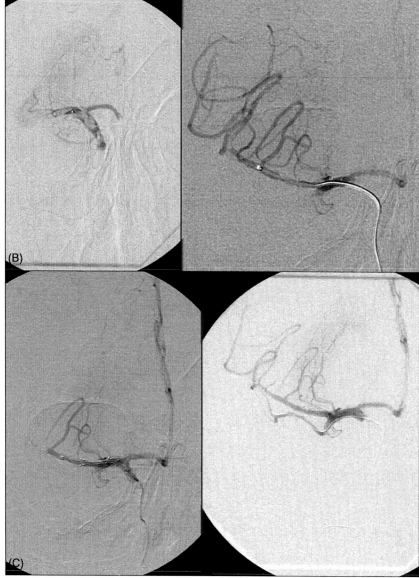

CS 4.2

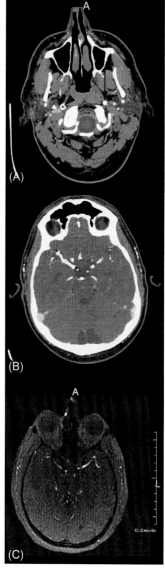

CS 4.3

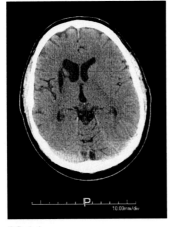

CS 4.4

Case study 5. Moyamoya disease, treated with the encephaloduroarteriosynangiosis procedure

A 25-year-old woman had cerebral palsy due to a perinatal right hemispheric stroke shown on CT scan (**CS 5.1**), and her MRA (not shown) suggested bilateral moyamoya vasculature.

Conventional angiography (**CS 5.2**)

The early phase study (left ICA injection) (A) shows prominent P1 and PCA anatomy (arrowhead) and an enlarged ophthalmic artery (arrows), with small arterial, telangiectatic anatomy in the region of the proximal MCA (encircled). The later phase (B) shows large proximal ACA anatomy, as well as several collateral routes directly connecting the distal ACA and PCA branches (arrowheads). Extensive extracranial external carotid artery–intracranial collateral segments have developed into the anterior circulation (right-hand side of images). An anteroposterior

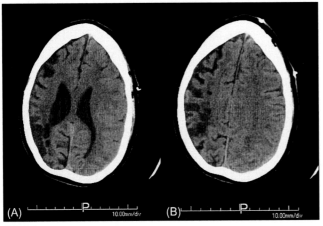

CS 5.1

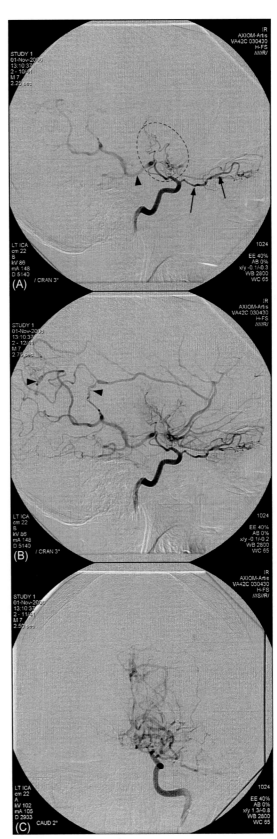

CS 5.2

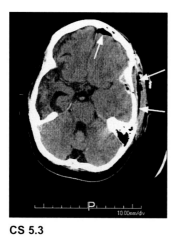

CS 5.3

view (C) documents markedly abnormal, small and large telangiectatic arteries encompassing the left ACA and MCA territories. A CT scan on the first postoperative day (**CS 5.3**) shows the region of the encephaloduroarteriosynangiosis, with air into the subdural and subgaleal spaces as well as the left anterior frontal lobe (arrows).

Follow-up angiography (**CS 5.4**)
Obtained 6 months following encephaloduroarteriosynangiosis, this study shows the development of external carotid artery (ECA)–MCA neovascular collateral blood supply.

The ECA injections shown are: (A) a lateral view of the left hemisphere and also anteroposterior views: subtracted (B, left) and unsubtracted (B, right) views; an ECA–MCA collateral pathway is marked (arrow). (The nasal turbines and orbital bones are present in the lower half of the images, marking the midline.)

Comments
This patient had bilateral moyamoya disease, presumed idiopathic, with a significant perinatal right hemispheric stroke. The decision to treat the left hemisphere with an encephaloduroarteriosynangiosis procedure was based on the plan to preserve the normal status of this dominant hemisphere, and the lack of an intact MCA recipient artery for a direct bypass procedure.

References

1. Adams H, Jr, Bendixen B, Kappelle L, *et al*. Classification of acute ischemic stroke: definition for use in a multicenter trial. *Stroke* 1993; **24**: 35–41.
2. Luscher T, Lie J, Stanson A, Houser O, Hollier L, Sheps S. Arterial fibromuscular dysplasia. *Mayo Clin Proc* 1987; **62**: 931–52.
3. Healton E, Mohr J. Cerebrovascular fibromuscular dysplasia. In: Barnett H, Mohr J, Stein B, Yatsu F, eds. *Stroke: Pathophysiology, Diagnosis, and Management*, 3rd edn. New York: Churchill Livingstone; 1998: 833–44.
4. Osborn A. Nonatheromatous vasculopathy. In: *Diagnostic Cerebral Angiography*, 2nd edn. Philadelphia, PA: Lippincott Williams & Wilkins; 1999: 341–58.

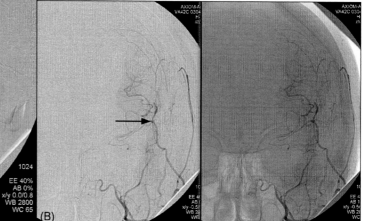

CS 5.4

5. Slovut D, Olin J. Fibromuscular dysplasia. *N Engl J Med* 2004; **350**: 1862–71.

6. Cloft H, Kallmes D, Kallmes M, Goldstein J, Jensen M, Dion J. Prevalence of cerebral aneurysms in patients with fibromuscular dysplasia: a reassessment. *J Neurosurg* 1998; **88**: 436–40.

7. Schievink W. Spontaneous dissection of the carotid and vertebral arteries. *N Engl J Med* 2001; **344**: 898–906.

8. Osborn A, Anderson R. Angiographic spectrum of cervical and intracranial fibromuscular dysplasia. *Stroke* 1977; **8**: 617–26.

9. Friedman W, Day A, Quisling J, *et al.* Cervical carotid dissecting aneurysms. *Neurosurgery* 1980; 7: 207–14.

10. Saver J, Easton J. Dissections and trauma of cervicocerebral arteries. In: Barnett H, Mohr J, Stein B, Yatsu F, eds. *Stroke: Pathophysiology, Diagnosis, and Management*, 3rd edn. New York: Churchill Livingstone; 1998: 769–86.

11. Mokri B. Cervicocephalic arterial dissections. In: Bogousslavsky J, Caplan L, eds. *Uncommon Causes of Stroke*. New York: Cambridge University Press; 2001: 211–29.

12. Fisher C, Ojemann R, Robertson G, *et al.* Spontaneous dissection of cervicocerebral arteries. *Can J Neurol Sci* 1978; **5**: 9–19.

13. Molina C, Alvarez-Sabin J, Schonewille W, *et al.* Cerebral microembolism in acute spontaneous internal carotid artery dissection. *Neurology* 2000; **55**: 1738–41.

14. Baumgartner R, Arnold M, Baumgartner I, *et al.* Carotid dissection with and without ischemic events: local symptoms and cerebral artery findings. *Neurology* 2001; **57**: 827–32.

15. Touze E, Randoux B, Meary E, Arquizan C, Meder J-F, Mas J-L. Aneurysmal forms of cervical artery dissection: associated factors and outcome. *Stroke* 2001; **32**: 418–23.

16. Schievink WI, Mokri B, O'Fallon WM. Recurrent spontaneous cervical-artery dissection. *N Engl J Med* 1994; **330**: 393–7.

17. Schievink WI, Mokri B, Piepgras DG, Kuiper JD. Recurrent spontaneous arterial dissections: risk in familial versus nonfamilial disease. *Stroke* 1996; **27**: 622–4.

18. Volker W, Besselmann M, Dittrich R, *et al.* Generalized arteriopathy in patients with cervical artery dissection. *Neurology* 2005; **64**: 1508–13.

19. Silverman IE, Wityk RJ. Transient migraine-like symptoms with internal carotid artery dissection. *Clin Neurol Neurosurg* 1998; **100**: 116–20.

20. Touze E, Gauvrit J-Y, Moulin T, Meder J-F, Bracard S, Mas J-L. Risk of stroke and recurrent dissection after a cervical artery dissection: a multicenter study. *Neurology* 2003; **61**: 1347–51.

21. Derex L, Nighoghossian N, Turjman F, *et al.* Intravenous tPA in acute ischemic stroke related to internal carotid artery dissection. *Neurology* 2000; **54**: 2159–61.

22. Georgiadis D, Lanczik O, Schwab S, *et al.* IV thrombolysis in patients with acute stroke due to spontaneous carotid dissection. *Neurology* 2005; **64**: 1612–14.

23. Lylyk P, Cohen J, Ceratto R, Ferrario A, Miranda C. Angioplasty and stent placement in intracranial atherosclerotic stenoses and dissections. *Am J Neuroradiol* 2002; **23**: 430–6.

24. Nadeau S. Diagnostic approach to central and peripheral nervous system vasculitis. *Neurol Clin* 1997; **15**: 759–77.

25. Biller J, Grau R. Cerebral vasculitis. In: Adams HP Jr, ed. *Handbook of Cerebrovascular Diseases*. New York: Marcel Dekker, Inc.; 2005: 653–72.

26. Calabrese L. Therapy of systemic vasculitis. *Neurol Clin* 1997; **15**: 973–91.

27. Weyand C, Goronzy J. Medium- and large-vessel vasculitis. *N Engl J Med* 2003; **349**: 160–9.

28. Zuber M. Isolated angiitis of the central nervous system. In: Bogousslavsky J, Caplan L, eds. *Uncommon Causes of Stroke*. New York: Cambridge University Press; 2001: 1–9.

29. Davis S. Temporal arteritis. In: Bogousslavsky J, Caplan L, eds. *Uncommon Causes of Stroke*. New York: Cambridge University Press; 2001: 10–17.

30. Singhal A, Koroshetz W, Caplan L. Cerebral vasoconstriction syndromes. In: Bogousslavsky J, Caplan L, eds. *Uncommon Causes of Stroke*. New York: Cambridge University Press; 2001: 114–23.

31. Reardon M, Mathews K. Moya moya disease. In: Adams HP Jr, ed. *Handbook of Cerebrovascular Diseases*. New York: Marcel Dekker, Inc.; 2005: 783–4.

32. Adams H, Jr. Moya-moya. In: Bogousslavsky J, Caplan L, eds. *Uncommon Causes of Stroke*. New York: Cambridge University Press; 2001: 241–57.

33. Yilmaz EMP, Bruno A, Lopez-Yunez A, Biller J. Moyamoya: Indiana University Medical Center experience. *Arch Neurol* 2001; **58**: 1274–8.

34. Chiu D, Shedden P, Bratina P, Grotta J. Clinical features of moyamoya disease in the United States. *Stroke* 1998; **29**: 1347–51.

35. Kuroda S, Hashimoto N, Yoshimoto T, Iwasaki Y. Radiological findings, clinical course, and outcome in asymptomatic moyamoya disease: results of multicenter survey in Japan. *Stroke* 2007; **38**: 1430–5.

36. Masuda J, Ogata J, Yamaguchi T. Moyamoya disease. In: Barnett H, Mohr J, Stein B, Yatsu F, eds. *Stroke: Pathophysiology, Diagnosis, and Management*, 3rd edn. New York: Churchill Livingstone; 1998: 815–32.

37. Suzuki Y, Negoro M, Shibuya M, Yoshida J, Negoro T, Watanabe K. Surgical treatment for pediatric moyamoya disease: use of the superficial temporal artery for both areas supplied by the anterior and middle cerebral arteries. *Neurosurgery* 1997; **40**: 324–30.

38. Kinugasa K, Mandai S, Kamata I, Sugiu K, Ohmoto T. Surgical treatment of moyamoya disease: operative technique for encephalo-duro-arterio-myo-synangiosis, its follow-up, clinical results, and angiograms. *Neurosurgery* 1993; **32**: 527–31.

39. Whitaker J. Management of moyamoya syndrome. *Arch Neurol* 2001; **58**: 132.

40. Ross R. Atherosclerosis—an inflammatory disease. *N Engl J Med* 1999; **340**: 115–26.

41. Krueger B, Okazaki H. Vertebral-basilar distribution infarction following chiropractic cervical manipulation. *Mayo Clin Proc* 1980; **55**: 322–32.

42. Fisher C, Ojemann R, Robertson G. Spontaneous dissection of cervico-cerebral arteries. *Can J Neurol Sci* 1978; **5**: 9–18.

Further reading

Bogousslavsky J, Caplan LR, eds. *Uncommon Causes of Stroke*. Cambridge University Press; 2001.

Osborn A. Nonatheromatous vasculopathy. In: *Diagnostic Cerebral Angiography*, 2nd edn. Philadelphia, PA: Lippincott Williams & Wilkins; 1999: 341–58.

Schievink W. Spontaneous dissection of the carotid and vertebral arteries. *N Engl J Med* 2001; **344**: 898–906.

Slovut D, Olin J. Fibromuscular dysplasia. *N Engl J Med* 2004; **350**: 1862–71.

Cervical Artery Dissection in Stroke Study. An international randomized clinical trial comparing anticoagulation to antiplatelet therapy for secondary stroke prevention in patients with cervical artery dissection has begun a feasibility stage. http://www.dissection.co.uk/

Resources for patients

Fibromuscular dysplasia

The Fibromuscular Dysplasia Society of America.
http://www.fmdsa.org
Fibromuscular Dysplasia, NINDS.
http://www.ninds.nih.gov/disorders/fibromuscular_dysplasia/fibromuscular_dysplasia.htm

Moyamoya disease

Moyamoya Disease, NINDS.
http://www.ninds.nih.gov/disorders/moyamoya/moyamoya.htm

Temporal arteritis

Vasculitis, including Temporal Arteritis, NINDS.
http://www.ninds.nih.gov/disorders/vasculitis/vasculitis.htm

Chapter 6

Therapies: The Management of Acute Ischemic Stroke and Secondary Stroke Prevention

Introduction

The rapidly evolving and increasing ability to treat AIS effectively is one of the most exciting topics in medicine. Acute stroke treatment is time-dependent so it is important to stress the need for stroke victims to reach the hospitals most able to offer the best combination of drug and device treatment(s). This means that regional stroke networks and efficient transfer processes will be key to increasing the number of people treated. This chapter addresses the state of acute treatments and secondary prevention for ischemic stroke.

Overview

Key variables influencing the viability of brain tissue during AIS include: **time, hemodynamics, tissue**, and **intervention** (*Table 6.1*).[1] Most of the effort to improve outcomes in ischemic stroke has focused on decreasing the time to treatment and pharmacologic or mechanical interventions for reperfusion or neuroprotection. More sophisticated assessment of hemodynamic issues, particularly collateral circulation, may influence what interventions are recommended at what point in time. Maximizing tissue viability through tight control of serum glucose and hypothermia is being evaluated.

The challenges of providing optimal treatment for every patient to improve clinical outcomes are significant:

1 *Time*. Although the healthcare systems in many countries are evolving to address acute stroke as a highest-level medical emergency, public awareness of stroke symptoms remains low. If stroke symptoms are not recognized or

patients not rapidly transported to 'stroke-ready' hospitals, then any efforts to develop treatments to improve stroke outcomes during the critical initial minutes-to-hours will be wasted. In the USA, Emergency Medical Services (EMS) are organized at the community and/or state-wide level making the early response to acute stroke patients highly variable. Benchmarks for hospital performance have been established to encourage rapid treatment on arrival.[2] The recommended time from door-to-computed tomography (CT) scan is 25 minutes, and from door-to-drug (intravenous (IV) tissue plasminogen activator (t-PA)) 60 minutes.

2 *Healthcare resources*. The capacity of individual hospitals to care for acute stroke varies widely. In the USA, national and regional quality improvement initiatives have led to formal certification/identification of acute 'stroke-ready' medical centers;[3] however, many hospitals lack adequate infrastructure and medical staff to meet all of the needs of acute stroke patients. Most likely, a two-tiered system will emerge with Primary Stroke Centers capable of rapid triage and administration of IV thrombolysis partnering with regional Comprehensive Stroke Centers that offer subspecialty neurovascular care, clinical trials, physician training programs, and endovascular (IA) treatments. The Joint Commission began certifying Primary Stroke Centers in the USA in 2004, and criteria for Comprehensive Stroke Centers have been published.[4]

3 *Stroke clinical trials*. The modern era of acute stroke clinical trials is in its infancy in regard to drug and device development and clinical trial design. Patient selection and outcomes can be based on clinical criteria alone or may include neuroimaging criteria. The pathophysiologic heterogeneity of stroke makes the assessment of outcomes even more challenging.[5]

Table 6.1 Factors for tissue viability in acute ischemic stroke

1. Time
- Acute Stroke Team, protocols → reduce time-to-treatment
- Public awareness → use of '911' EMS systems
- *Impact*: speed time to starting acute therapies

2. Hemodynamics
- *Collateral circulation*: circle of Willis; leptomeningeal
- Extracranial and intracranial stenoses
- *Measure*: neuroimaging to define, perfusion CT/MRI studies
- *Impact*: manipulate systemic blood pressure, acute occlusive lesions

3. Tissue
- Local metabolic, hemostatic, vascular, structural changes secondary to ischemia
- *Measure*: age, gender, serum glucose, temperature, blood pressure, oxygenation
- *Impact*: correcting treatable variables that may impact upon brain tissue viability (e.g., hyperthermia, hyperglycemia, coagulability)

4. Intervention
- Reperfusion tactics, neuro/cytoprotection
- *Impact*: IV/IA thrombolysis, devices for vessel recanalization

Adapted from Warach.[1]

4 *Complexity of cerebral ischemia.* Understanding of the biology of cerebral ischemia, which is the basis for new drug and device development, continues to evolve. The time-dependent cascade of acute focal ischemia is illustrated (**6.1**).[6] Drugs that interrupt or slow the ischemic cascade may interact with only one of the various steps. Ischemia affects not only neurons (constituting <5% of the cells in cerebral gray matter) but also astrocytes and other glial cells supporting neurons, the axons of neurons (which relay signals to other cells), and the microvessels that supply oxygen and nutrients.[7] Treatments that target this entire 'neurovascular unit' rather than simply neurons may be more effective in treating acute ischemic brain injury (**6.2**).[7]

Treatment for acute ischemic stroke

The modern era of treatments for AIS was ushered in by clinical trials that began in the 1980s and early 1990s. Two major therapeutic approaches have been studied since the early trials were conducted:

- **Reperfusion treatments** include IV or IA drugs and endovascular devices aimed at the recanalization of occluded intracranial and extracranial arteries. IV t-PA was approved for the treatment of AIS within 3 hours of onset of symptoms in the USA in 1996.[8] The MERCI Retriever was approved for the removal of clots from intracranial and extracranial cerebral arteries within 8 hours of stroke symptoms onset in 2004 (**6.3; case study 1**).[9] A second endovascular thrombectomy device, the Penumbra Stroke System, was similarly approved by the Food and Drug Administration (FDA) in 2008 for its aspiration mechanism.[10]
- **Neuroprotective agents** or devices are meant to maintain optimal tissue viability in the ischemic penumbra. No pharmacologic agent has been shown to be effective. Trials of hypothermia and infrared laser to test potential for neuroprotection are currently in progress.[11]
- The scope of established and putative treatments for AIS is shown in *Table 6.2*.[11] The stage is set for an explosion in treatment modalities during the upcoming decades.[6,7,12]

Reperfusion treatment and time

Time is brain! For every minute stroke is left untreated, an estimated 1.9 million neurons are destroyed.[13] The benefit of IV t-PA has been demonstrated to wane through the 3-hour window.[14] However, subsequent pooled analysis of three major clinical trials suggests that the time window of effectiveness for IV t-PA may actually be as long as 4.5 hours.[15] Recent clinical trials evidence from the European study group subsequently went on to prove that IV t-PA is efficacious for AIS within this 3 to 4.5-hour time window.[16]

IA treatments, initially catheter-delivered thrombolytic agents, such as pro-urokinase[17,18] directly address the arterial clot responsible for AIS. In addition to drugs, the catheter itself and other devices such as balloon angioplasty, flexible stents, and clot retrieval devices can be used to manipulate thrombus and recanalize vessels. Successful outcomes with IA treatment may occur well beyond the traditional 3-hour

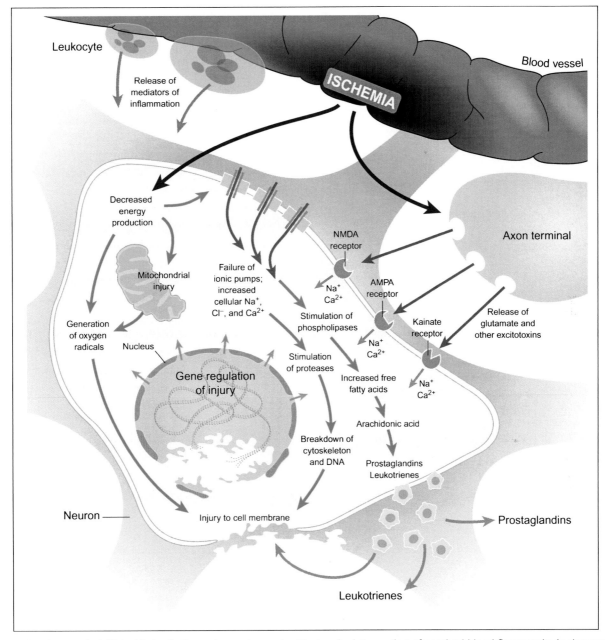

6.1 The molecular events initiated in brain tissue by acute cerebral ischemia. Interruption of cerebral blood flow results in decreased energy production, which in turn causes failure of ionic pumps, mitochondrial injury, activation of leukocytes (with release of mediators of inflammation), generation of oxygen radicals, and release of excitotoxins. Increased cellular levels of sodium, chloride, and calcium ions result in stimulation of phospholipases and proteases, followed by generation and release of prostaglandins and leukotrienes, breakdown of DNA and the cytoskeleton, and ultimately, breakdown of the cell membrane. Alteration of genetic components regulates elements of the cascade to alter the degree of injury. AMPA denotes α-amino-3-hydroxy-5-methyl-4-isoxazole propionic acid and NMDA *N*-methyl-D-aspartate. Adapted with permission from Brott *et al.*[6]

time window for IV t-PA. Timeframes of 6–8 hours for anterior circulation strokes and 12–48 hours for posterior circulation strokes have been reported in case series and formal clinical trials (Chapter 4, **case study 2**).[12]

The two leading endovascular approaches are IA thrombolysis and the MERCI clot retrieval device (this chapter, **case study 1**; Chapter 3, **case study 1**). IA thrombolysis has limited randomized clinical trial data to support its

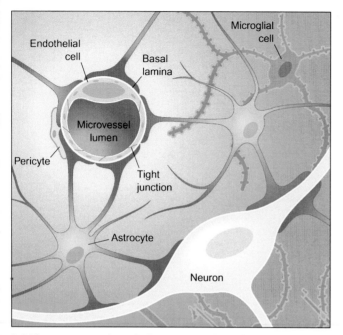

6.2 The neurovascular unit. A conceptual framework, the neurovascular unit is comprised of neurons, the microvessels that supply them, and their supporting cells. Cerebral microvessels consist of the endothelium (which forms the blood–brain barrier), the basal lamina matrix, and the end-feet of astrocytes. Microglial cells and pericytes may also participate in the unit. Communication has been shown to occur between neurons and microvessels through astrocytes. Adapted from del Zoppo.[7]

efficacy.[18,19] Current guidelines recommend IA thrombolysis for selected patients who have major stroke of <6 hours duration due to occlusions of the MCA and who are otherwise not candidates for IV t-PA and for patients with contraindications (e.g., recent surgery) to the use of IV thrombolysis;[20] however, criteria for patient selection and evaluation of optimal IA treatments are subjects of ongoing investigation.[19]

The potential advantages of IA thrombolysis over IV t-PA include: direct angiographic visualization of the lesion responsible for AIS; the ability to mechanically disrupt the thrombus with guidewire and catheter; improved recanalization rates for selected proximal lesions of higher thrombus burden (e.g., basilar,[21] proximal MCA,[22] and distal ICA occlusions[23]); lower dose of thrombolytic agent (e.g., 5–20 mg IA t-PA, versus a maximal IV t-PA dose of 90 mg); and the longer time windows. The MERCI clot retrieval device also enables direct analysis of the pathogenesis of AIS, when thromboembolic material is retrieved for pathologic study (**6.3**).[9,24] The potential barriers to the widespread use of endovascular approaches are their limited availability at acute care hospitals in most countries and the additional time, often 1–2 hours, to prepare such interventional procedures.

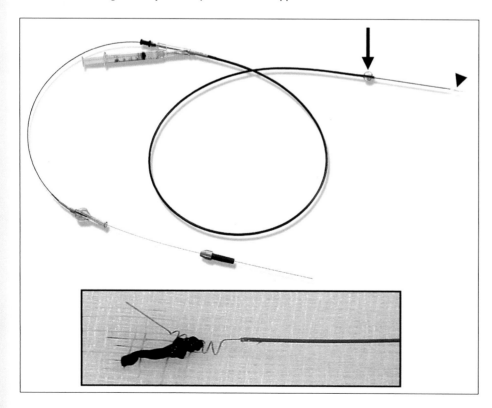

6.3 The MERCI clot retrieval device.[9] The earlier-generation clot retrieval device consists of a flexible helical snare (arrowhead) that uncoils beyond and into the thrombo-occlusive lesion (see inset), and a balloon (arrow) that enables proximal protection, to prevent blood flow from fragmenting and embolizing the ensnared clot up into the cerebral vasculature. Image published with permission, courtesy of Concentric Medical, Inc.

Table 6.2 Therapeutic modalities for reperfusion therapy during acute ischemic stroke

Fibrinolytic agents
- Established: IV t-PA
- Novel, experimental: tenecteplase, desmoteplase, reteplase, microplasmin

Glycoprotein IIb/IIIa antagonists
- Abciximab, tirofiban

Combined pharmacological approaches

a. Lytics and antithrombotics
   (i) Examples (in preliminary trials): IV t-PA + tirofiban; reteplase + abciximab; eptifibatide + t-PA; argatroban (direct thrombin inhibitor) + t-PA

b. Lytics and neuroprotectants
   (i) Hypothermia
   (ii) Magnesium (in field), with in-hospital reperfusion

c. Lytics and vasoprotectants
   (i) NXY-059 (spin trap agent) ± IV t-PA

d. Sonothrombolysis
   (i) 2-MHz continuous ultrasound monitoring + t-PA

Endovascular mechanical treatments
- Intra-arterial fibrinolysis
- Mechanical disruption of occlusive material
- Endovascular thrombectomy

Note: The above list includes drugs and devices that have been trialed, rejected, and/or approved in clinical studies. t-PA, tissue plasminogen activator.
Adapted from Molina *et al.*[12]

Combination modalities

Some of the combined modalities for treatment studied to date are listed in *Table 6.2*. The development of multimodal approaches combining drugs and devices is not dissimilar from those employed for acute coronary syndromes.[11,25] Key challenges with acute pharmacologic and endovascular interventions in the brain versus the heart are: (1) greater technical difficulty in accessing intracranial arteries with endovascular devices due to smaller, more tortuous vessels; (2) the susceptibility to reperfusion hemorrhage in the brain; and (3) limited accessibility to interventional specialists to perform endovascular procedures for AIS. In the USA, for example, hundreds of hospitals are capable of performing IA treatments for acute coronary syndromes, while only a few dozen are well-staffed with neurointerventionalists to treat AIS around the clock.

Neuroimaging

Modern neuroimaging has revolutionized acute stroke treatment by helping clinicians to more accurately and rapidly select patients best suited for emergent interventions.

Multimodal MRI and CT imaging protocols, developed only in the past decade, help identify patients most likely to benefit from reperfusion and direct treatments based on lesion-specific data. Neuroimaging differentiates AIS from acute hemorrhage, detects very early ischemia, quantifies and delineates irreversibly infarcted core tissue from salvageable penumbra, demonstrates areas of hemorrhagic transformation, and identifies large vessel occlusions and stenoses. All of this information can be rapidly obtained in 5–20 minutes.[12] The resultant data indicate the degree of collateral circulation, a critical variable in eventual infarct size. Strong collateral circulation (direct, via the circle of Willis, and indirect, via adjacent leptomeningeal supply) can keep a large area of penumbral tissue viable for an extended period of time, while patients with poor collaterals are less likely to do well even with early recanalization. The neuroimaging data enable patient selection based upon an individualized, physiologic 'tissue clock' rather than a fixed chronologic clock.[12]

The concept of the 'mismatch model' discussed in Chapter 1 to assess areas of brain viability based on perfusion MRI and CT techniques is gaining credibility. In this model, a core (irreversible) infarct is surrounded by a region of salvageable ischemic penumbra, and an adjacent region of benign oligemia.[26] Modern clinical trials have begun to incorporate real-time neuroimaging data into their patient selection and outcomes data. Current research is utilizing functional MRI and CT imaging in an effort to select patients with viable ischemic tissue who could benefit from recanalization beyond 3 hours. These newer neuroradiologic techniques may identify those patients who may be assisted by reperfusion and other treatments as well as those who cannot be helped (**case study 2**) and who could even potentially be harmed.

Management of acute ischemic stroke

Acute stroke is 'brain shock.' The part of the brain that is affected lacks blood supply and, therefore, oxygen and glucose. The goal is to reperfuse as quickly as possible and resuscitate 'shocked (stunned) brain.' Guidelines on the standard of care for patients with AIS are published periodically by the American Stroke Association (*Table 6.3*).[20] Ample clinical trials evidence also has demonstrated that stroke patients' outcomes are improved with care in dedicated stroke units, largely by averting post-stroke medical complications (e.g., deep vein thrombosis, aspiration).[27]

In cases of massive hemispheric stroke, most typically involving the entire territory of the MCA, the development of malignant edema results in herniation syndromes with high early mortality rates. Hemicraniectomy (removal of the skull on one side of the head, with duraplasty) is sometimes recommended as a life-saving tactic (**case study 3**).[28] Recently, a pooled analysis of three randomized controlled European trials documented a strong benefit of this approach in patients <60 years of age with malignant MCA territory infarction.[29] Patients with large infarcts of the cerebellar hemisphere, usually in the territory of the posterior inferior cerebellar artery, may similarly face a high early mortality from brainstem compression, yet also have encouraging outcomes with surgical decompression of the posterior fossa (Chapter 4, **4.3**).

It is likely that acute stroke treatment will always be time-dependent, with the best outcomes resulting from the earliest interventions paired with meticulous medical management in dedicated stroke units. It is also likely that treatment decisions will be based more and more on an individual patient's cerebrovascular physiology rather than strict time limits. The approach will be to permanently open the occluded vessel with drugs and/or devices as rapidly as possible while protecting vulnerable cells with neuroprotective drugs or devices.

Secondary prevention of stroke

Once an ischemic stroke has occurred, the patient is at an increased risk for a second event, especially over the ensuing days or weeks.[30] The first step in secondary prevention is to determine the cause of the stroke, if possible. If there is a mechanical cause that can be corrected such as significant

---

Table 6.3 Basic management of patients with acute ischemic stroke[20]

- *Body position*: the patient should be supine in the bed.
- *Oxygen*: all stroke victims should initially be placed on supplemental oxygen.
- *Blood pressure*: both elevated and low blood pressure are associated with poor outcomes after stroke.[41] There are no definite guidelines for blood pressure levels immediately after AIS. Ischemic brain loses its autoregulation so the oxygen available for tissue becomes completely dependent on perfusion pressure which in turn is dependent on mean arterial blood pressure. Prior to reperfusion, blood pressure should remain high. Blood pressure no higher than 185/110 is the recommended level for administration of IV t-PA, and 180/105 for the initial 24 hours after IV t-PA treatment. After reperfusion, there is the risk of reperfusion injury (i.e., hemorrhage and edema), particularly at higher blood pressures. If pressures drop, particularly with worsening of clinical status, normotonic fluids without glucose should be used for resuscitation. Pressors can be considered in some cases, especially to encourage collateral blood flow in patients with defined proximal occlusive disease.
- *Hyperglycemia*: patients with elevated blood glucose following AIS have poorer outcomes.[42] In general, the desired blood glucose levels are 80–140 mg/dl.
- *Temperature*: fever should be treated to normothermia. Hypothermia is being tested to see if it improves outcomes from AIS.
- *Antithrombotic agents*: the standard timing of antithrombotic agents is 24 hours after the administration of IV t-PA or other reperfusion modalities. Patients who are not candidates for thrombolysis or other reperfusion treatments should be administered aspirin within 48 hours after onset of the stroke.

AIS, acute ischemic stroke; t-PA, tissue plasminogen activator.

carotid stenosis or patent foramen ovale (PFO), then procedures to correct the lesion should be considered in some cases. There are established data to support carotid endarterectomy over medical management in surgical candidates who have a >70% stenosis of the symptomatic carotid artery.[31] The benefits and risks of carotid stenting versus carotid endarterectomy are being evaluated in clinical trials.[32] Transcatheter devices and increasingly less-invasive open surgical approaches to close PFO are available, but have not yet been shown to be superior to medical management.[33,34] Vertebral and intracranial artery stenoses can be treated with angioplasty and stenting if the patient remains symptomatic on optimal medical treatment, and clinical trials will address the proper role of the use of stents in this setting.[35,36]

Table 6.4 Recommended goals for stroke risk factors[31,43]

Blood pressure	<120/70
Total cholesterol	<200
Low-density lipoprotein	<100 (in diabetics, <70)
Smoking cessation	
Maximum alcohol	2 drinks per day for males; 1 drink per day for females
Exercise 5 days per week	
Normal body weight	

Table 6.5 Options for antiplatelet therapy[31,39]

- Aspirin alone at doses of 81–325 mg daily has been shown to be effective in multiple trials
- Clopidogrel at 75 mg daily is effective (CAPRIE)[44]
- The combination of clopidogrel and Aspirin is not more effective than either agent alone, and the combination produces excess bleeding (CHARISMA[45], MATCH[46]).
- The combination of low dose aspirin and extended release dipyridamole is more effective than Aspirin alone (ESPS-2[47], ESPRIT[48]).
- The combination of low dose aspirin and extended release dipyridamole is as effective as clopidogrel in secondary stroke prevention (PRoFESS[49]).'

Identification of stroke risk factors is the next important step in secondary prevention. Hypertension, diabetes, smoking, and hyperlipidemia are the major risk factors, but obesity, inactivity, excess use of alcohol, and stress may also be important. *Table 6.4* summarizes recommended goals for risk factor management. The 'big three' of secondary stroke prevention are antithrombotic treatment, antihypertensive agents, and lipid-lowering treatment.[31] Recent randomized clinical trials have extensively addressed the importance of controlling these risk factors. Efforts to further drive down levels of blood pressure and low-density lipoprotein appear to be increasingly effective in stroke prevention.[37,38]

The last step in effective secondary prevention is selection of antithrombotic treatment.[39] In general, treatment with warfarin is the most effective way to prevent recurrent cardioembolic stroke. In most cases the International Normalized Ratio (INR) should be 2–3, with the exception of patients with artificial cardiac valves in which the INR should be 2.5–3.5. Warfarin is no better than aspirin in preventing recurrent stroke in patients with intracranial disease, and has a higher risk.[40] For all other types of strokes, including those caused by small vessel disease, antiplatelet treatment is recommended. *Table 6.5* summarizes the options for antiplatelet treatment and the trials supporting their use.

Case studies

Case study 1. Endovascular recanalization of a carotid T lesion

History
A 51-year-old woman with a history of hypertension and dyslipidemia presented on the morning of admission with right-sided hemiparesis. She was last seen well at 05:30, and subsequently found down by family member at 07:00.

Timeline
Emergency department
- 05:30–7:00, symptoms onset.
- 07:43, EMS dispatched.
- 08:10, Emergency Department arrival.
  - *Exam*: she could follow some commands, but was densely dysarthric with non-fluent aphasia, left gaze preference, right hemiparesis and neglect.
  - NIHSS score = 14 points.

- 08:30–8:40, head CT and CT angiography were obtained (**CS 1.1**):
  - a hyperdense left MCA sign was observed consistent with left M1 occlusion (A)
  - a normal left ICA bifurcation (B), but coronal intracranial images (C) show diminished flow in the distal left ICA as well as the M1 and A1 segments consistent with a carotid T occlusion
  - the CT perfusion study was incompletely processed, but a time-to-peak map suggests substantial left hemispheric ischemia (blue region) (D)
  - owing to the uncertainty of time from symptoms onset and the large clot located at the carotid T (likely to be unresponsive to IV t-PA alone), consent was obtained from the patient's husband for IA revascularization procedures.
- 09:10, anesthesia was started, with elective intubation.

Endovascular procedure

1 *Diagnostic angiography* (**CS 1.2**):
  - left ICA injection, posterior lateral views, shows mild cervical FMD (A,B), with a tortuous, redundant proximal cervical segment (A, arrows) as well as an acute intracranial occlusion (arrowheads), just above the level of the anterior choroidal artery
  - right ICA injection, anteroposterior (AP) projection, shows good cross-filling via the anterior communicating artery into the left A1 segments and distal ACA branches, with some leptomeningeal collateralization into the left MCA territory (arrows) (C).

2 *Interventional treatment* (**CS 1.2**, continued):
- 10:30, angiography during the procedure shows progressive reopening of the distal M1/proximal M2 occlusion, AP view (D).
  - A single pass of the MERCI LX device resulted in excellent recanalization; the post-procedure AP (E) and a comparison of lateral views, pre-procedure (F, left) versus post-procedure (F, right).

3 *Pathology and post-treatment MRI scan* (**CS 1.3**):
  The procedure aspirated a <2-cm thrombus, shown attached to the MERCI LX device (A), and alone (B). The pathologist's evaluation of the clot identified only fibrin and red blood cells.
- 12:16, transfer to Neuroscience ICU.
- 15:15, extubated.
- 16:45, brain MRI shows a small lesion on diffusion-weighted (arrowhead) (C) and FLAIR (D) sequences, with a normal intracranial MRA (E).

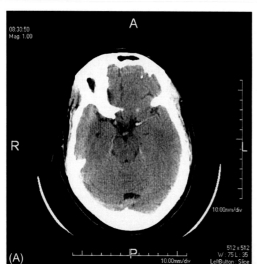

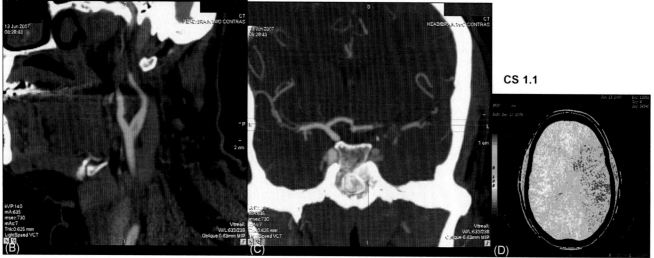

CS 1.1

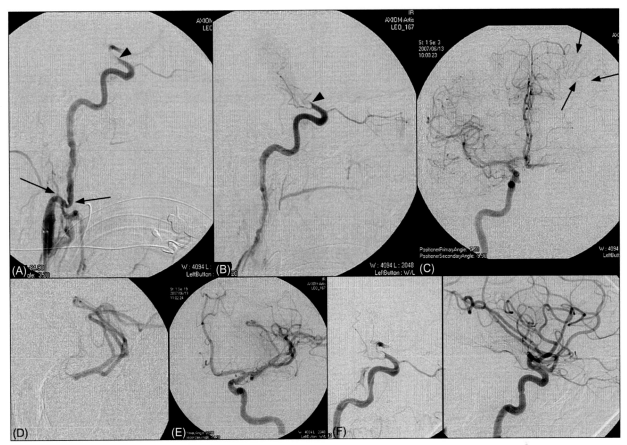

CS 1.2

Hospital course
- **Hospital day (HD) 2**, NIHSS score = 0 points.
- **HD3**, a TEE study showed a PFO with an interatrial septal aneurysm, and spontaneous right-to-left shunting. Anticoagulation was started.
- **HD4**, a lower-extremity venous Duplex ultrasound scan showed acute thrombus involving one posterior tibial vein and one peroneal vein in the left leg.
  - Laboratory studies were significant for elevated serum low-density lipoprotein, 116 mg/dl; and elevated C-reactive protein, 1.46 (normal range, 0–0.49 mg/dl).
- **HD5**, discharge to rehabilitation, on warfarin and statin treatment with no neurologic deficits.

Comments

This patient made an outstanding recovery from early endovascular recanalization. Her relatively low NIHSS score for a carotid T lesion probably reflected excellent native collateral circulation. The stroke etiology was likely paradoxical thromboembolism from a deep vein thrombosis,

via a PFO. Secondary stroke prevention in this setting is controversial, with newer transcatheter and less invasive open surgical methods to close the PFO.[33,34] With identification of a deep vein thrombosis, warfarin for the first several months is an appropriate antithrombotic agent. Another risk factor to consider over the long-term is this patient's cervical FMD.

Case study 2. Intravenous thrombolysis with a 'matched' computed tomography perfusion study
History

A 75-year-old man with a history of tobacco use and hypertension presented to a local hospital with a left hemispheric stroke syndrome.

Timeline and hospital course
- 08:30, symptoms onset.
- 0 h 30 min, arrival at local hospital.
- 0 h 50 min, non-contrast head CT scan (not shown).
- 1 h, contact regional stroke center facility via 1-800 Stroke Hotline.

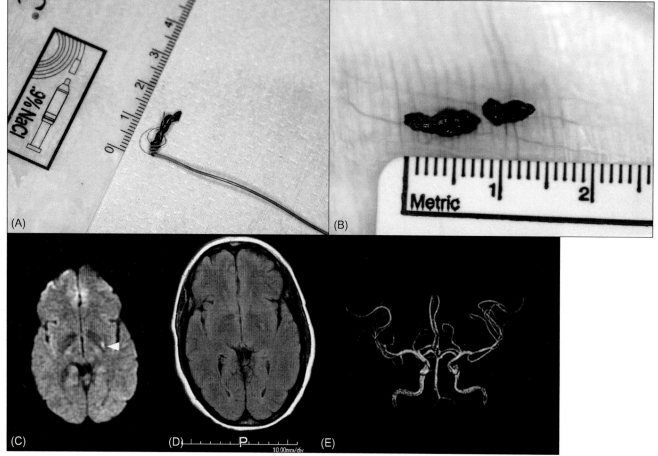

CS 1.3

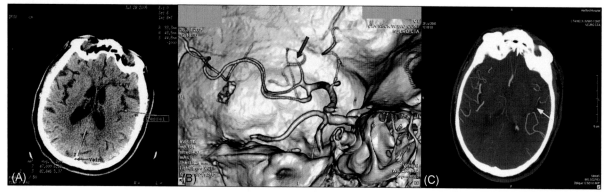

CS 2.1

- 2 h, bolus and infusion of IV t-PA started at local hospital.
- 3 h, arrival at regional stroke center:
  - initial NIHSS score = 22 points.
- 3 h 50 min, head CT scan (**CS 2.1A**):
  - CT angiography documents an M3 occlusion of the left MCA, shown on reconstructed three-dimensional study (B) (pink arrow) and maximum intensity projection (C) (yellow arrow).
- 4 h, CT perfusion (**CS 2.2**):
  - processing of the CT scan, and decision, with the neurointerventional team, to not pursue an endovascular procedure. The low-density lesion most prominent on the cerebral blood flow map (a black–dark blue region)

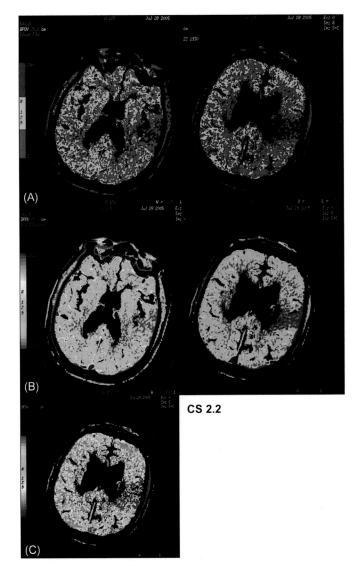

CS 2.2

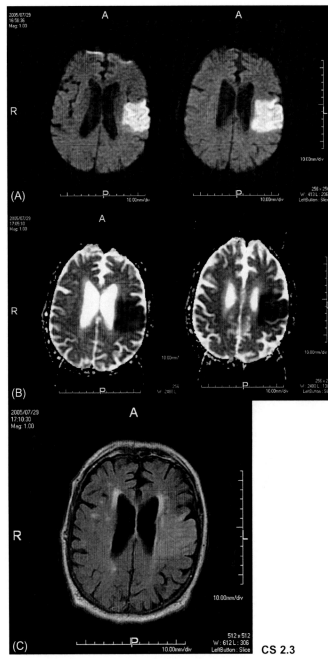

CS 2.3

(A) matches that on the cerebral blood volume (blue) (B) and mean transit time maps (blue) (C), indicating no viable penumbra (a 'matched' pattern).

- **HD2**
  - MRI (**CS 2.3**) on the next day, diffusion-weighted image sequences (A) and apparent diffusion coefficient map (B), corroborated the lesion on the previous day's CT perfusion scan as a wedged-shaped infarct. The final lesion on the FLAIR sequence (C) is comparable with the area of low cerebral blood volume (**CS 2.2B**).

- **HD6**
  - The patient is discharged to rehabilitation with a predominantly expressive aphasia, and some early return of right leg strength
  - Hospital discharge NIHSS score = 12 points.

Comments

The initial clinical evaluation upon arrival at the tertiary care center suggested a wide area of ischemia involving an occlusion in the first- or second-order left MCA. However, CT angiography showed a more peripheral third-order (M3) occlusion, and the largely matched cerebral blood flow and cerebral blood volume lesions suggested no ischemic penumbra at risk that would benefit from an endovascular procedure.[12,26,50,51]

Despite a relatively high initial NIHSS score (>20 points), the Stroke Team decided not to offer additional treatments beyond IV thrombolysis. The subsequent MRI scan confirmed a peripheral frontoparietal lesion. The patient's early recovery during the acute hospitalization was encouraging and validated this clinical decision.

Case study 3. Hemicraniectomy for the malignant middle cerebral artery syndrome

History and exam

A 56-year-old man was hospitalized for pneumonia. Two days later, he developed a right hemispheric stroke syndrome, with dysarthria, left hemiplegia, and hemineglect.

Timeline

HD1   Acute stroke symptoms onset.

HD3   Transfer to the regional stroke center. Serial head CT scans (**CS 3.1**):

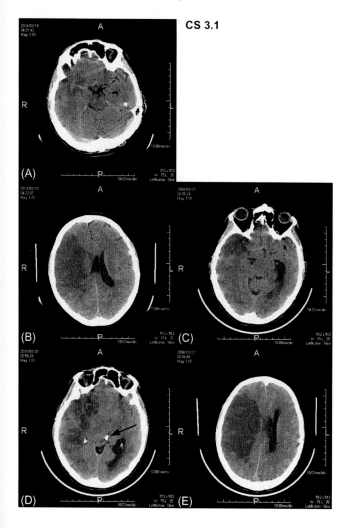

CS 3.1

HD4   Admission head CT scan shows an early large right MCA stroke (A,B).

- *Exam*: alert and conversant; left hemianopia and hemineglect; dense left hemiplegia. NIHSS score = 16 points.
- Neurosurgery consult to consider hemicraniectomy.

HD6   Deteriorating mental status prompted repeat head CT scan (C–E):

- Extensive right uncal herniation has markedly obscured the entire posterior fossa, with pressure on the midbrain and trapping of the contralateral left ventricle (C), midline shift of the calcified pineal gland (arrow) (D), and well-delineated MCA-territory infarct with subfalcine herniation (E).

HD6   **Hemicraniectomy (CS 3.2)**. The patient's wife was consented for this procedure.

- Following a large curvilinear incision from the anterior tragus back toward the occipital bone and to the midline of scalp (A, left), burr holes are made (A, right), and a wide skull bone window is removed (B).
- The exposed brain shows signs of elevated intracranial pressure, with engorged superficial veins (C). Following this craniotomy, the dura is closed with the addition of fascia latae from the scalp (arrows) (D).

HD7   **Postoperative day 1**, Neuroimaging (**CS 3.3**):

- head CT scan shows severe edema, pushing brain beyond the former skull margin, with some normalization toward midline. A single transaxial view (A) and composite views (B,C) demonstrate how the infarcted brain extends beyond the skull margin. A postoperative lateral skull film shows the stapled wound (D), and three-dimensional CT scan shows a postoperative AP view (E).

HD15   Transfer to acute rehabilitation.
Day 60 Recovery:

- Walking 80–100 feet, holding a quad cane in the right hand.
- Left shoulder subluxation on plain X-ray.

Day 84 Cranioplasty procedure (CS 3.4).

- The skull bone is replaced 3 months later (A): reconstructive surgery to encompass the region where the temporalis muscle was removed.
- Post-cranioplasty FLAIR MRI sequence (B,C). Note that there are small areas of apparently intact brain tissue within the large right MCA stroke.

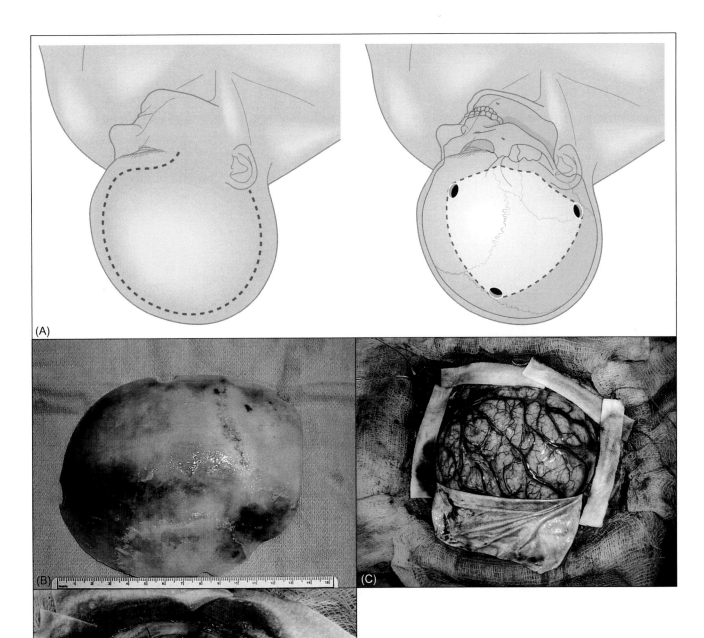

- The patient following cranioplasty, with a widened palpebral fissure and mild lower facial paresis on the left (D).
- NIHSS score = 7 points, largely from residual left hemiparesis.

Day 104 Returns home from assisted living facility. Ambulating with quad cane.

A second patient, aged 51, underwent craniotomy for a malignant right MCA syndrome, and returned to the stroke clinic 1 year later, ambulatory, but with significant left hemiparesis (**CS 3.4E**). Note the left ankle–foot orthosis, and flexor posturing of the left hand.

CS 3.2

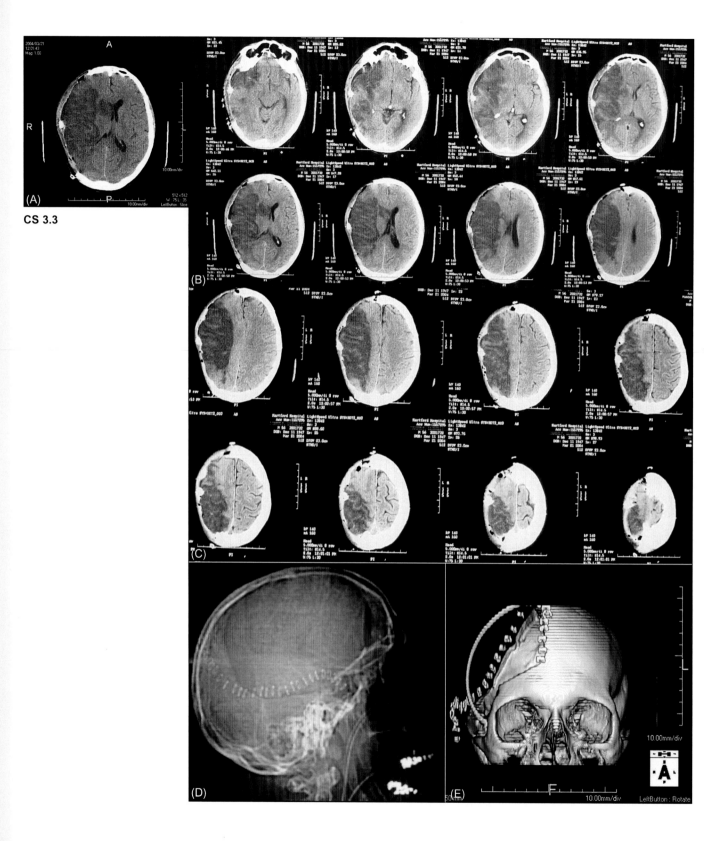

CS 3.3

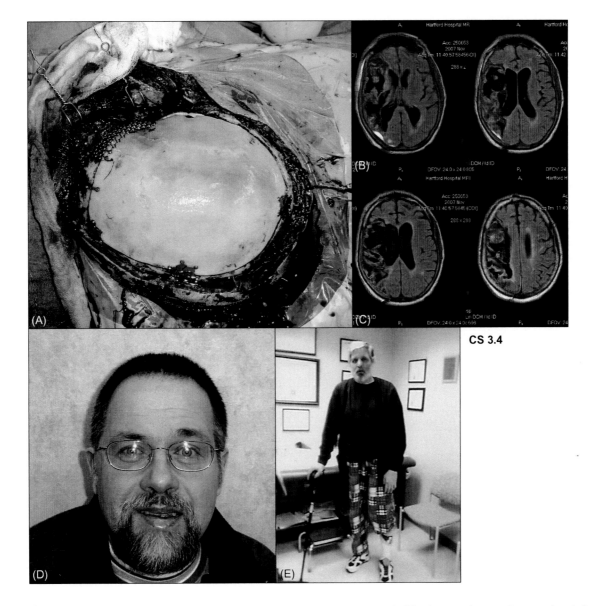

CS 3.4

Comments

Hemicraniectomy works. In an analysis of three randomized clinical trials, the procedure benefited not only survival but also short-term outcomes.[27] The time-to-randomization in this analysis was 45 hours, in order to begin the surgical procedure within 48 hours. Patient selection included an NIHSS score >15 points, with a diminished level of consciousness. The short-term survival was improved from 29% in the medical (placebo) arm, versus 78% in the treatment (surgical) arm. The number needed to treat to result in a single favorable outcome at 12 months, defined as modified Rankin Scale of ≤4 points, was two patients.

Key observations about these data are: (1) most case series and clinical trials work restrict the procedure to patients ≤60 years of age; (2) an excellent outcome from

this life-threatening stroke may be defined by the ability to return to an ambulatory state, as the patients presented here did; and (3) the decision to intervene should be made within the first 12–48 hours, soon after acute treatments (e.g., IV t-PA and endovascular approaches) have been attempted yet before significant progression toward uncal herniation. In practice, hemicraniectomy is typically recommended for the treatment of non-dominant hemisphere strokes, but can also be considered for highly selected patients with left hemispheric stroke.

Some of the functional recovery seen with hemicraniectomy may relate to the salvaging of brain tissue within the ischemic penumbra (CS 3.4B,C). The patches of spared brain presumably avert pressure necrosis against the adjacent skull when that tissue acutely swells.

References

1. Warach S. Tissue viability thresholds in acute stroke: the 4-factor model. *Stroke* 2001; **32**: 2460–1.

2. Tilley B, Lyden P, Brott T, Lu M, Levine S, Welch K. Total quality improvement method for reduction of delays between emergency department admission and treatment of acute ischemic stroke. *Arch Neurol* 1997; **54**: 1466–74.

3. Alberts M, Hademenos G, Latchaw R, *et al.* Recommendations for the establishment of primary stroke centers. *JAMA* 2000; **283**: 3102–19.

4. Alberts M, Latchaw R, Selman W, *et al.* Recommendations for comprehensive stroke centers: a consensus statement from the Brain Attack Coalition. *Stroke* 2005; **36**: 1597–618.

5. Fisher M. Recommendations for advancing development of acute stroke therapies: Stroke Therapy Academic Industry Roundtable 3. *Stroke* 2003; **34**: 1539–46.

6. Brott T, Bogousslavsky J. Treatment of acute ischemic stroke. *N Engl J Med* 2000; **343**: 710–22.

7. del Zoppo G. Stroke and neurovascular protection. *N Engl J Med* 2006; **354**: 553–5.

8. National Institute of Neurological Disorders and Stroke rt-PA Stroke Study Group. Tissue plasminogen activator for acute ischemic stroke. *N Engl J Med* 1995; **333**: 1581–7.

9. Smith W, Sung G, Starkman S, *et al.*, for the MERCI Trial Investigators. Safety and efficacy of mechanical embolectomy in acute ischemic stroke: results of the MERCI Trial. *Stroke* 2005; **36**: 1432–40.

10. McDougall C, Clark W, Mayer T, *et al.* The Penumbra Stroke Trial: safety and effectiveness of a new generation of mechanical devices for clot removal in acute ischemic stroke [abstract]. International Stroke Conference (New Orleans) 2008; LB4.

11. Konstas A-A, Choi J, Pile-Spellman J. Neuroprotection for ischemic stroke using hypothermia. *Neurocrit Care* 2006; **4**: 168–78.

12. Molina C, Saver J. Extending reperfusion therapy for acute ischemic stroke: emerging pharmacological, mechanical, and imaging strategies. *Stroke* 2005; **36**: 2311–20.

13. Saver J. Time is brain-quantified. *Stroke* 2006; **37**: 263–6.

14. Marler JR, Tilley BC, Lu M, *et al.* Early stroke treatment associated with better outcome: The NINDS rt-PA Stroke Study. *Neurology* 2000; **55**: 1649–55.

15. Hacke W, Donna G, Fieschi C, *et al.* Association of outcome with early stroke treatment: pooled analysis of ATLANTIS, ECASS, and NINDS rt-PA stroke trials. *Lancet* 2004; **363**: 768–74.

16. Hacke W, Kaste M, Bluhmki E, *et al.* Thrombolysis with alteplase 3 to 4.5 hours after acute ischemic stroke. *N Engl J Med* 2008; **359**: 1317–29.

17. Furlan A, Higashida R, Katzan I, Abou-Chebl A. Intra-arterial thrombolysis in acute ischemic stroke. In: Lyden P, ed. *Thrombolytic Therapy for Stroke*. Totowa, NJ: Humana Press; 2001: 175–95.

18. Furlan A, Higashida R, Wechsler L, *et al.* Intra-arterial prourokinase for acute ischemic stroke. The PROACT II Study: a randomized controlled trial. *JAMA* 1999; **282**: 2003–11.

19. Mattle H. Intravenous or intra-arterial thrombolysis? It's time to find the right approach for the right patient [editorial]. *Stroke* 2007; **38**: 2038–40.

20. Adams H, Jr, del Zoppo G, Alberts M, *et al.* Guidelines for the early management of adults with ischemic stroke: a guideline from the American Heart Association/American Stroke Association Stroke Council, Clinical Cardiology Council, Cardiovascular Radiology and Intervention Council, and the Atherosclerotic Peripheral Vascular Disease and Quality of Care Outcomes in Research Interdisciplinary Working Groups. *Stroke* 2007; **38**: 1655–711.

21. Lindsberg P, Mattle H. Therapy of basilar artery occlusion: a systematic analysis comparing intra-arterial and intravenous thrombolysis. *Stroke* 2006; **37**: 922–8.

22. Agarwal P, Kumar S, Hariharan S, *et al.* Hyperdense middle cerebral artery sign: can it be used to select intra-arterial versus intravenous thrombolysis in acute ischemic stroke? *Cerebrovasc Dis* 2004; **17**: 182–90.

23. Zaidat O, Suarez J, Santillan C, *et al.* Response to intra-arterial and combined intravenous and intra-arterial thrombolytic therapy in patients with distal internal carotid artery occlusion. *Stroke* 2002; **33**: 1821–7.

24. Marder V, Chute D, Starkman S, *et al.* Analysis of thrombi retrieved from cerebral arteries of patients with acute ischemic stroke. *Stroke* 2006; **37**: 2086–93.

25. Rogalewski A, Schneider A, Ringelstein E, Schabitz W-R. Toward a multimodal neuroprotective treatment of stroke. *Stroke* 2006; **37**: 1129–36.

26. Kidwell CS, Alger JR, Saver JL. Beyond mismatch: evolving paradigms in imaging the ischemic penumbra with multimodal magnetic resonance imaging. *Stroke* 2003; **34**: 2729–35.

27. Stroke Unit Trialists Collaboration. How do stroke units improve patient outcomes? A collaborative systematic review of the randomized trials. *Stroke* 1997; **28**: 2139–44.

28. Schwab S, Steiner T, Aschoff A, *et al.* Early hemicraniectomy in patients with complete middle cerebral artery infarction. *Stroke* 1998; **29**: 1888–93.

29. Vahedi K, Hofmeijer J, Juettler E, *et al.* Early decompressive surgery in malignant infarction of the middle cerebral artery: a pooled analysis of three randomised controlled trials. *Lancet* 2007; **6**: 215–22.

30. Rothwell P, Warlow C. Timing of TIAs preceding stroke: time window for prevention is very short. *Neurology* 2005; **64**: 817–20.

31. Sacco R, Adams R, Albers G, *et al.* Guidelines for prevention of stroke in patients with ischemic stroke or transient ischemic attack. *Stroke* 2006; **37**: 577–617.

32. Furlan A. Carotid-artery stenting—case open or closed? [editorial]. *N Engl J Med* 2006; **355**: 1726–9.

33. Adams H, Jr. Cardiac disease and stroke: will history repeat itself? *Mayo Clin Proc* 2006; **81**: 597–601.

34. Kizer J, Devereux R. Patent foramen ovale in young adults with unexplained stroke. *N Engl J Med* 2005; **353**: 2361–72.

35. Fiorella D, Levy E, Turk A, *et al.* US multicenter experience with the Wingspan stent system for the treatment of intracranial atheromatous disease: periprocedural results. *Stroke* 2007; **38**: 881–7.

36. Zaidat O, Klucznik R, Chaloupka J, *et al.* An NIH-funded multicenter registry on the use of the Wingspan intracranial stent for high-risk patients with symptomatic intracranial arterial stenosis [abstract]. International Stroke Conference (San Francisco) 2007; LB3.

37. PROGRESS Group. Randomised trial of a perindopril-based blood-pressure-lowering regimen among 6105 individuals with previous stroke or transient ischaemic attack. *Lancet* 2001; **358**: 1033–41.

38. The Stroke Prevention by Aggressive Reduction in Cholesterol Levels (SPARCL) Investigators. High-dose atorvastatin after stroke or transient ischemic attack. *N Engl J Med* 2006; **355**: 549–59.

39. Albers G, Amarenco P, Easton J, Sacco R, Teal P. Antithrombotic and thrombolytic therapy for ischemic stroke: The Seventh ACCP Conference on Antithrombotic and Thrombolytic Therapy. *Chest* 2004; **3**: S483–512.

40. Chimowitz MI, Lynn MJ, Howlett-Smith H, *et al.* Comparison of warfarin and aspirin for symptomatic intracranial arterial stenosis. *N Engl J Med* 2005; **352**(13): 1305–16.

41. Castillo J, Leira R, Garcia M, Serena J, Blanco M, Davalos A. Blood pressure decrease during the acute phase of ischemic stroke is associated with brain injury and poor stroke outcome. *Stroke* 2004; **35**: 520–6.

42. Baird T, Parsons M, Phanh T, *et al.* Persistent poststroke hyperglycemia is independently associated with infarct expansion and worse clinical outcome. *Stroke* 2003; **34**: 2208–14.

43. Chobanian A, Bakris G, Black H, *et al.* Seventh report of the Joint National Committee on prevention, detection, evaluation, and treatment of high blood pressure (JNC 7—Complete Version). *Hypertension* 2003; **42**: 1206–52.

44. CAPRIE Steering Committee. A randomised, blinded, trial of clopidogrel versus aspirin in patients at risk of ischaemic events (CAPRIE). *Lancet* 1996; **348**: 1329–39.

45. Bhatt D, Fox K, Hacke W, *et al.* Clopidogrel and aspirin versus aspirin alone for the prevention of atherothrombotic events. *N Engl J Med* 2006; **354**: 1706–17.

46. Diener H-C, Bogousslavsky J, Brass L, *et al.* Aspirin and clopidogrel compared with clopidogrel alone after recent ischaemic stroke or transient ischaemic attack in high-risk patients (MATCH): randomised, double-blind, placebo-controlled trial. *Lancet* 2004; **364**: 331–7.

47. Diener H, Cunha L, Forbes C, Sivenius J, Smets P, Lowenthal A. European Stroke Prevention Study 2. Dipyridamole and acetylsalicylic acid in the secondary prevention of stroke. *J Neurol Sci* 1996; **143**: 1–13.

48. The ESPRIT Study Group. Aspirin plus dipyridamole versus aspirin alone after cerebral ischaemia of arterial origin (ESPRIT): randomised controlled trial. *Lancet* 2006; **367**: 1655–73.

49. Sacco R, Diener H-C, Yusuf S, *et al.* Aspirin and extended-release dipyridamole versus clopidogrel for recurrent stroke. *N Engl J Med* 2008; **359**: 1238–51.

50. Lev M, Segal A, Farkas J, *et al.* Utility of perfusion-weighted CT imaging in acute middle cerebral artery stroke treated with intra-arterial thrombolysis: Prediction of final infarct volume and clinical outcome. *Stroke* 2001; **32**: 2021–8.

51. Wintermark M, Reichhart, Thiran JP, *et al.* Prognostic accuracy of cerebral blood flow measurement by perfusion computed tomography, at the time of emergency room admission in acute stroke patients. *Ann Neurol* 2002; **51**: 417–32.

Further reading

Adams H, Jr, del Zoppo G, Alberts M, *et al.* Guidelines for the early management of adults with ischemic stroke: a guideline from the American Heart Association/American Stroke Association Stroke Council, Clinical Cardiology Council, Cardiovascular Radiology and Intervention Council, and the Atherosclerotic Peripheral Vascular Disease and Quality of Care Outcomes in Research Interdisciplinary Working Groups. *Stroke* 2007; **38**: 1655–711.

del Zoppo G. Stroke and neurovascular protection. *N Engl J Med* 2006; **354**: 553–5.

Lyden P. *Thrombolytic Therapy for Stroke*. Towana, NJ: Humana Press; 2001. This textbook provides a superb overview of the development of IV and IA thrombolysis for AIS, along with case studies.

Sacco RL, Adams R, Albers G, *et al.* Guidelines for prevention of stroke in patients with ischemic stroke or transient ischemic attack. *Stroke* 2006; **36**: 577–617.

Warach S. Tissue viability thresholds in acute stroke: The 4-factor model. *Stroke* 2001; **32**: 2460–1.

INDEX